MW00848592

Secrets of
Street Survival—
ISRAELI
STYLE

Secrets of
Street Survival–
ISRAELI STYLE
Staying Alive in a
Civilian War Zone

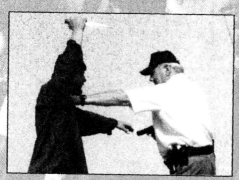

Eugene Sockut

Paladin Press
Boulder, Colorado

Also by Eugene Sockut:

Secrets of Gunfighting Israeli Style (video)

Secrets of Street Survival—Israeli Style:
Staying Alive in a Civilian War Zone
by Eugene Sockut

Copyright © 1995 by Eugene Sockut

ISBN 10: 0-87364-819-6
ISBN 13: 978-0-87364-819-6
Printed in the United States of America

Published by Paladin Press, a division of
Paladin Enterprises, Inc.
Gunbarrel Tech Center
7077 Winchester Circle
Boulder, Colorado 80301 USA
+1.303.443.7250

Direct inquiries and/or orders to the above address.

Visit our Web site at www.paladin-press.com

Contents

Introduction 1

1 The Correct Mind-Set 3

2 Know Thine Enemy 61

3 Street Weapons—"Cold" 89

4 Street Weapons—"Hot" 153

5 Gun Rigs for the Street 209

6 The Street 249

7 In the Vehicle 279

8 Securing Your Home from the Streets 325

9 Survival in Riots 359

Warning

Some of the techniques and drills, armed and unarmed, that are depicted in this book are extremely dangerous. It is not the intent of the author or publisher to encourage readers to attempt any of these techniques and drills without proper professional supervision and training. Attempting to do so can result in severe injury or death. Do not attempt any of these techniques or drills without the supervision of a certified instructor.

The author and the publisher disclaim any liability from any damage or injuries of any type that a reader or user of information contained within this book may encounter from the use of said information. This book is *for information purposes only.*

Introduction

We live in frightening times, some say cataclysmic times—times when street survival becomes an increasingly needed skill. The world has undergone massive changes since the so-called "normal" decade of the 1950s, when life was so much simpler. Street survival in those days meant keeping clear of well-known bad neighborhoods. Most people didn't lock the doors of their homes and most certainly not their cars. Crime, if present, was mostly of the petty type, without violence. Murder was so uncommon it was the stuff headlines were made of. An old double-barreled shotgun loaded with bird shot or a .32-caliber automatic filled with round-nose jacketed bullets was considered state-of-the art by most civilians and was usually more than adequate for protection of home and hearth.

Alas, those days are as dead as the proverbial dodo bird. Today, we face the crazies: armed drug gangs who would rather kill than rob you, dope addicts who commit murder and then forget the reason they did it in the first place, seemingly insane sex killers who murder their innocent victims in bizarre rituals of devil worship. And suddenly, rising like a phoenix from the ashes, Islamic fundamentalist fanatics, spiritually fueled from Iran, doctrinal brothers of the infamous Moros of the Philippine Insurrection, seeking the slaughter of the accursed infidel in the twisted belief that the cool waters and lovely damsels of a heavenly paradise await their self-inflicted martyrdom for Allah.

Paladin Press encouraged my idea about bringing to its worldwide readership the secrets of street survival learned here in Israel, a nation where street survival is a way of life (or death). The lessons learned here are not set forth as being the only way to "skin a cat," nor are they considered the ultimate wisdom on the subject, for there are no absolutes in the field of self-defense. Those of us who are self-defense specialists by profession strive to be objective. We are constantly learning and many times publicly eating the words we've spoken and written. And that is how it should be, since our craft is an art and not a science.

I believe the Israeli experience is unique, acting as a test bed of the immediate future, a future that seems to be slowly spiraling down into a dark abyss where all the fears that nightmares are made of suddenly spring to life.

It is my contention the world faces historical dislocations that will be triggered by monetary collapse. This will cause severe and unprecedented social, political, and economic chaos. Already, depression and inflation are rearing their ugly heads higher and higher. This will prove fertile ground for street terror and crime. I hope that governments will rise to the occasion and protect us all. However, I have always believed that real security begins at home. We are the ultimate masters of our fate. We are the captains of our ship.

This book represents a lifetime of study and experimentation and is an extract of the best ideas that I have garnered from those who have seen the wolf and conquered him. The study and experimentation continues as I approach my sixtieth year, for the threat to the innocent changes daily and a keen eye must be kept open so as to conquer it. Sitting at my desk in the pine-forested hills outside of the eternal city of Jerusalem, I work with this thought in mind and humbly offer you this book: *Secrets of Street Survival—Israeli-Style: Staying Alive in a Civilian War Zone.*

Chapter One

The Correct Mind-Set

*I*n Shakespeare's play *Hamlet*, there is a famous scene wherein the Prince of Denmark stares at a human skull and asks a very basic question of survival: "To be or not to be, that is the question. Whether it is nobler in the mind to suffer the slings and arrows of outrageous fortune or to take up arms against a sea of troubles and by opposing end them?"

These lines could also have been written to express the deep psychological dilemma some people face when confronted with deadly force and who suddenly realize that they are mentally unprepared.

The individual who is psychologically unprepared to use deadly force in a life-or-death confrontation is almost certainly doomed to failure, since he faces not one but two adversaries—himself and his enemy, an enemy who almost certainly has no qualms about taking his life. The old adage "he who hesitates is lost" applies in spades when street survival is the order of the day.

Having now worked in weapons training for more than three decades, I'm still amazed at the number of individuals who purchase a handgun and then proclaim to all and sundry: "I don't want to kill anybody; I just want to scare them." These individuals undoubtedly feel that their enemies share the same humanistic philosophy. They almost assuredly do not. Crime statistics prove this contention.

Street criminals, terrorists, individuals berserk on drugs, as well as psychopaths have already made a decision to kill. Some have decided not to be apprehended and will even charge against a drawn pistol rather than risk prison. One has no leeway against such predators, and they expect and give no quarter.

Many have tried to understand why some people seem to be natural-born victims. Why do they almost insist on being victims? Psychiatrists claim such an attitude is at least partially caused by something they call denial.

DENIAL

Denial is based on the human trait of self-delusion. This psychological concept can be described in layman's terms as: "If I make believe this terrible thing is not happening to me, then it will cease to be happening and go away."

Many individuals simply refuse to believe in the imminence of approaching injury or in the possibility of their own death at the hands of some evil perpetrator. Many tend to view human behavior through their own eyes and, since they would not be capable of committing cold-blooded murder, cannot accept the fact that others do such things without hesitation.

In Nazi-occupied Europe, a vast network of murder factories gassed millions of innocent people. We tend to focus in on the Jews, since they were the principal target group, but besides the 6 million Jews who were murdered, there were also millions of others who were Christians, Allied prisoners of war, Gypsies, the handicapped, and so on. In the end, Hitler planned to depopulate Eastern Europe of tens of millions of Poles, Slavs, and other ethnic groups.

One of the most common human traits shared by many

of these victims was denial—the refusal to believe that the horrible catastrophe that was unfolding before their very eyes was actually happening. They learned the hard way that evil lurks on this earth. It did then, and it most certainly does today.

Lecturing to Israelis, I make a point of telling them of the phenomena of denial and use a brutal form of shock technique, relating vivid pictures of brutal murders, substituting word pictures for the actual experience of a personal attack, attempting to wake them out of the world of denial by showing them mentally into the world of the street, where cruel predators roam. I find it amazing that even here in Israel, after the Holocaust, there are still many who practice denial.

Case Study: Jerusalem Bus Attack

Recently, I was paid a visit by an individual who went through the experience of a terrorist attack and has since resolved "never again." Like many police officers, he learned that the weapon on his belt was not put there to weigh him down but was an instrument of reality.

Debriefing

Jonathan (ex-U.S. Ranger, street cop, and SWAT team member) and I debrief Thomas, age 35, a recent immigrant from North America.

Sequence of Action

A busy street. Thomas drives his car behind a bus in north Jerusalem and hears three shots. The bus at the top of a hill loses control and swings to the side. Thomas: "I knew a terrorist attack was taking place." The cars around the bus drive away. Thomas pulls over, draws a .45-caliber STAR PD auto, and jacks a jacketed ball round into the chamber. (He does not carry any spare loaded magazines.)

Suddenly, the front door of the bus opens and a body falls halfway out. Thomas says he is approximately 50 yards from the bus. A man carrying a short M16 rifle jumps out of the bus and runs from it carrying his rifle in a "military fashion."

This leads Thomas to the false conclusion that the man is an Israeli undercover police officer. He believes the man with the M16 is chasing after a terrorist armed with a handgun who he thinks fired on the bus from a nearby hill.

Thomas jumps out of his car and sees that the man he had mistaken for an undercover police officer seems surprisingly calm as people run around him screaming "terrorist!" Thomas wants to shoot, but he sees an old house and innocent Arabs milling about. They begin to understand what is happening and wail in fear. Thomas is afraid he will hit them if he fires at the terrorist, who is now only some 20 yards away. He also realizes for the first time the monumental error of not having any spare loaded magazines. He asks himself, "What do I do after round number six?" Thomas yells, "Get down!" to the innocent bystanders. He wants to fire a warning shot (still unfortunately done in the Mideast) but decides not to do this since he fears a bloodbath if he alarms the terrorist. Then he hears more shots coming from the direction of the bus. He stares down at his pistol and thinks to himself, "I am going to die. I don't have enough ammo."

He sees people running in shock from the bus. Some, recent Russian immigrant women, are crying and screaming hysterically.

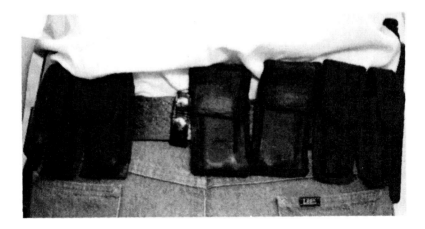

FOR THE CORRECT MIND-SET: Carrying enough loaded magazines on you helps alleviate concerns of running out of ammo in a firefight.

Thomas aims again and then stops, realizing he almost definitely will hit someone behind the terrorist since his marksmanship ability is not very high. Thomas runs a few steps and is then confronted by an angry Israeli woman, who shouts, "Why are you running?! Shoot the S.O.B.!"

Thomas turns and is shocked to find himself in a Mexican standoff with the terrorist who has the handgun. The terrorist (Thomas knows this now) armed with the M16 screams something to the other terrorist. They run to an opening in a stone wall 15 yards away from Thomas and both disappear from view.

Thomas walks back to the bus and sees the body of the man shot in the head. He is lying in the street, wounded. He is not an Israeli, nor is he the bus driver, as Thomas had previously surmised, but an Arab from Gaza.

Soldiers and police arrive and ask Thomas for a description of the two terrorists, who by now have escaped through some backyards and kidnapped an Israeli woman in her car. They have reportedly been spotted driving at high speed toward the south section of Jerusalem.

The police order Thomas to stay with them, since they still cannot ascertain if the two kidnappers are the same two

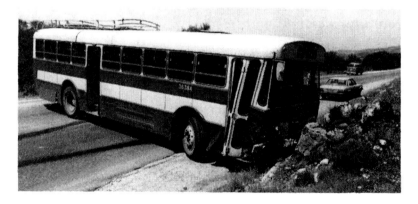

AMBUSHED BUS: This particular bus was first disabled by oil poured onto the road, which caused the driver to lose control and crash. It was then attacked.

terrorists from the bus incident or members of some other gang operating in the area. A report comes over the radio of a shoot-out between police and the two kidnappers. Thomas goes with the police to the site of the shoot-out. He reports to us, "There was nothing to identify, since the two bodies were burnt to a crisp."

Jeanette Kadosh-Dayan lay dead in the street, shot by her kidnappers and thrown from her car. They were the two terrorists.

Terror Timetable

7 A.M.—Egged bus No. 25 pulls away from Neveh Yaacov, a neighborhood in north Jerusalem.

7:13—Two terrorists board the bus carrying bags filled with weapons and explosives.

7:35—A police car passing nearby reports that gunfire is heard coming from the bus.

7:35—The terrorists kidnap Jeanette Kadosh-Dayan outside her office and take her car. Massive army and police reinforcements stream into the area to search for the terrorists.

8:10—The kidnap vehicle races toward an army roadblock in south Jerusalem. Kadosh-Dayan is shot by the terrorists and thrown out of the speeding car. Soldiers open fire. The car races out of control for 20 yards, smashes into a tree, and explodes into flames.

More Details Emerge

Passenger Olga Khaikov, 42, dies of gunshot wounds to her head when she is shot by the terrorists on the bus. She was a recent Jewish immigrant from Russia and the mother of an 11-year-old daughter.

Jeannette Kadosh-Dayan, 39, was the mother of four. She was buried in a funeral attended by hundreds.

Unarmed (he could not afford a gun) bus driver David Yom-Tov, 33, was wounded in the thigh by a terrorist when he attempted to overpower the gunman and prevent him from slaughtering the passengers. He was assisted in this by another Israeli man from Neveh Yaacov whose identity is not known.

The man who was shot in the head and fell from the bus was Salah Othman, 22, a Hamas Moslem fundamentalist. It is still not clear who shot him, whether he was a third terrorist, or if his presence on the bus was a coincidence. He is in very serious condition. (File still open.)

The terrorists had left bombs in the area of the bus. All were later disarmed by police sappers.

The two dead terrorists were identified as members of the Izadin Kassem military wing of Hamas.

Some Interesting Consequences

A few years ago, Thomas was called upon to identify a friend who was murdered with four others, ambushed from a rooftop in Hebron by terrorists using Carl-Gustav submachine guns and grenades.

Another one of the murdered men was my friend Eli Ha-Zeev, a former American Vietnam war veteran who had served two tours as a "tunnel rat." An excellent professional soldier who had just visited me a few days before his murder, Eli carried a S&W Model 39 in those tunnels and had lost a thumb to a Vietcong RPG. He was one of my shooting instructors in the Israel Defense Forces (IDF). The terror attack took place under the window of the apartment where my mother lives in Jerusalem.

The bus driver and passenger who attacked the terrorists barehanded were cited for bravery. Their intervention undoubtedly saved the lives of many passengers. I have learned the bus driver will be presented with a pistol.

....

STREET SURVIVAL LESSONS

1)   *Never needlessly endanger others.* Both Jonathan and I agree that Thomas acted correctly since he did not have a clear field of fire, lacked proper training in the use of his weapon, lacked tactical know-how, and did not have confidence in his ability to hit his target.

2) *Don't practice denial.* Prior to facing the reality of a terrorist attack, Thomas had practiced denial. Even though he purchased a handgun (after viewing his dead friend's body), he never really believed he would ever have to use it.

3) *Have enough ammunition on hand.* The lack of even one spare loaded magazine (denial once again) caused Thomas to be fearful about running out of bullets in a firefight. These thoughts were swirling around in Thomas' mind, causing him to hesitate. He froze and became a mere bystander.

4) *Accept the use of deadly force.* You must accept the unpleasant fact that you may be forced to take human life. Repetitive exercises alone will not guarantee that you will perform. They must be based on a correct mind-set based on your prior acceptance of the use of deadly force.

Summary

Almost any game plan is better than no game plan. We cannot be absolutely certain how any of us will react in any and all circumstances, but forewarned is certainly forearmed. Thomas now knows that to have a gun does not make one a gunfighter. He is diligently working to change that. Like hundreds of police officers and citizens before him who have faced death in the street and somehow survived, he now has a good chance of becoming a formidable gunfighter. He now accepts the fact that the ability "to be or not to be" lies mostly in his own hands.

Thomas is now practicing with his weapon in a serious combat shooting program and has vowed never again to be caught without some scenario plan when facing deadly force. He also has vowed never to be without spare ammunition and has purchased extra magazines for his STAR PD.

THINK LIKE AN ALLEY CAT

Many times I am asked by people, "How can I walk in the street and avoid becoming a victim?" My pat answer is to observe an alley cat foraging for food in a garbage bin or sunning himself on top of a wall. Suspicion is its middle name. It trusts no one. The alley cat is on full alert even when squinting at you through half-closed eyes. Make a move toward it and it is off for parts unknown. That's how alley cats have survived all these centuries in a constantly changing and hostile environment.

Alley cats assume anything living is an enemy, and even when proven wrong, still keep a high state of alert just in case. They know that the closer any living creature gets to them the more the danger increases. That's why they stare so intently, watching to see if you are closing the gap between you and them. These are difficult creatures to sneak up on, these masters of street survival.

Some of my students complain, "I can't live that way. I can't spend my life waiting to be attacked." My pat answer is, "We are responsible for how we choose to live and, many times, how we choose to die. If you choose to be protected only by the laws of mathematical possibilities, you have a 50/50 chance of not ever facing a criminal encounter. But if you do, remember, you called the shots—you 'didn't want to live that way.'"

We cannot be on the street and act as if we were in our living room, safely behind locked doors and windows. The safe artificial environment we have constructed for ourselves has no relationship to the street. Out on the street we wander into the real world, a world filled with predators. Out there, any person, even one who looks utterly harmless, can be a mortal danger to your continued existence. Here in Israel, seemingly harmless-looking women walking in the street have pulled long, razor-sharp butcher knives and attacked unsuspecting individuals with deadly results. Looks can deceive. The notorious Boston Strangler gained entry into unsuspecting women's apartments by pretending to be a good-natured repairman. He looked harmless. He wouldn't have fooled an alley cat.

Danger doesn't always look like danger. Evil doesn't always look like evil. We have been brought up on horror movies, and most of us think people who do bad things look bad. This has not been the case in real life. When asking the neighbors of some mass murderer what kind of person he was, it's almost routine to hear, "Oh, he was such a nice, quiet man, always helpful and friendly. I just can't believe he'd ever hurt a fly. I'm in a state of shock. Did he really run a gas chamber? I don't believe it." Chances are our nice old man wouldn't have fooled our suspicious old alley cat, but he sure can fool naive, trusting souls.

I must have a tenth-generation group of cats around my farm here in the Judean Hills outside of Jerusalem. Every noon when I go to feed my dogs, I make sure they get fed, too. (They help keep the poisonous vipers away.) To this day, I can't quite pick one up, even though they purr around my legs at feeding time. Bend down toward them, and they are off and running. Their natural instinct to survive is very strong, and they will never knowingly place themselves in jeopardy by having blind trust.

Case Study: Desert Justice

Probably one of the most natural-born survivalists I've ever met (thinks like a cat) is Daniel, an Israeli man of the desert.

Daniel is an Israeli who lives in a particularly isolated desert area that is smack up against the Jordanian border. He tells me of the times when that border was not as quiet as it is at this writing. The following is that interview.

E.S.: You told me you lived in a little world of peace and tranquillity in a small area of desert some 3 kilometers by 3 kilometers where you herded your flocks of sheep. How could you survive in such an environment, living alone with your wife in a cave while guerrilla war was raging all around you?

D: I learned years ago that predators don't like to hunt people who hunt predators. Having people piss in their pants when they see you is a good way to insure a tranquil existence. I simply scared the hell out of those who wanted to kill me.

E.S.: How did you accomplish that? You were all alone against the many. One Israeli against hundreds.

D: Not by very nice methods, not things most people would understand, at least people from the West. However, the people of the desert understand life and death. I simply made it crystal clear that when they came over that particular area of border they were entering my world, and in my world, if you come in peace, you live, but if you come looking for trouble, you suffer and sometimes die.

For example, if some infiltrator came over the border looking for trouble and I felt in a generous mood, I simply cut off one of his ears and then put him up on my hanging tree.

E.S.: Hanging tree?

D: It was a lonely desert acacia tree. I'd lift him up into its gnarled and twisted branches and dry him out for a few days. Sooner or later someone would infiltrate across the border and visit with me. I did have some friends on the other side. We'd eat lunch under that tree, never once looking up at who was hanging in it. It would have been impolite to do that until we finished our Turkish coffee and then my guest would point over his head, still not looking up and ask, "What about him?" At this we would look up and see what was up there. It usually was someone with a blue tongue sticking out of his mouth, hanging quite peacefully. Then I'd ask: "Do you want him?" They always did, and I'd cut him down. I obtained quite a collection of ears from under that tree.

E.S.: Quite a novel way of maintaining the peace.

D: But, effective.

E.S.: You mentioned one particular sheik who was a very close friend.

D: He was a real man, something that people from the West haven't seen for a long time. A leader—feared, bright, and tough as hell.

E.S.: You killed him.

D: I had no choice, not if I wanted to live. I'm not proud of it. We were alike in a way, though I came from the West. It was sort of like an Indian fighter of the American West who killed the noble savage who he felt was superior to most men he ever knew. I'm not proud of that, killing him, no sir. He was a real man. A king of his tribe.

E.S.: Why did that happen? What made you kill him?

D: I was told by certain people—people I respected for their professionalism—that the Jordanian government didn't like me and that tribe having good, friendly relations. They didn't like him bringing other sheiks across the border to my area and having Passover and other Jewish holiday meals in my cave. They wanted it stopped, so they jailed some of his close relatives and then told him much worse would happen if he didn't come across the border and kill me.

It wasn't much longer before one of his men came and told me the sheik wanted to see me at sundown. It was then that I knew the secret information I obtained about him wanting to kill me was true. He was a man of the desert. He knew the rules.

E.S.: I don't understand.

D: Night is death out in the desert. Out on the sands, there are no police. Make one mistake and you're dead. I suspected an ambush. I knew that if I was trusting, made one mistake, I would have my throat slit. Out on the desert, if I'm not sure, and it's night, I prefer to kill my enemy. That's why I'm alive today. I'm alive and he's dead. But I'm not proud of it.

E.S.: What happened?

D: We [Daniel and the sheik's messenger] went on a trail, a trail that was getting darker and darker as the sun set in the distance. Suddenly, someone came out of the side of the trail. I fired. He was dead before he hit the ground. His man ran off in panic. I looked down. It was my friend, the sheik.

E.S.: What did you do then?

D: I melted into the dark and waited. Soon they came for his body and carried him across the border. I watched from a hill as his body was passed over the hands of hundreds. They screamed, wailed, grieving in a frenzy. They pulled him limb from limb. I grieved with them. I'm not proud I had to kill him. No, sir. It was the hardest thing I ever did. In a way, the sheik and I were victims in a war neither of us wanted. But it was him or me, and I'm alive to tell the tale.

STREET SURVIVAL LESSONS

1) *Think like an alley cat.* Be alert; trust no one you have objective cause to be suspicious of.

2) *Looks can deceive.* Don't be fooled. A harmless-looking person can kill. This is made much easier when you have let your defenses down, lowered your level of suspicion, watered down your instinct for survival. Daniel has a very strong survival instinct. He'll reach a ripe old age.

COLOR CODE WARNING SYSTEM

Over the years I have watched numerous color code warning systems develop from the original military one, the so-called "color codes of danger" developed by the U.S. Marines during World War II and the campaign against the Japanese in the Pacific.

CONDITION WHITE: You do not perceive the remote possibility of danger. You are unprepared and relaxed.

CONDITION YELLOW: Relaxed awareness of your immediate environment, which, though seemingly benign, does have some element of potential danger.

CONDITION ORANGE: You are suddenly alerted to a potential unknown danger. You react accordingly.

CONDITION RED: You are plunged into an actual violent situation with a dangerous opponent.

CONDITION BLACK: An extreme situation is in progress, and you may be fighting for your very life.

Many experts use the color code system or slight variations of it for civilian use. I beg to differ. Though the system has worked in the military context, I believe it is now inadequate as far as civilian street survival is concerned. The days of bad and good neighborhoods are gone. The days of suspicious-looking characters so easy to identify in Hollywood films are gone (if they ever really existed). We live in an age of rampant, growing crime. Old boundaries have vanished. Over one-third of all North American city dwellers have been victims of crime. This has spilled over into the suburbs, where this figure is fast being approached. Crime is rising by leaps and bounds. At least half of the people now living in North America will fall victim to some type of crime sometime in the future.

During the so-called Rainbow Rebellion that took place after the first Rodney King verdict in Los Angeles, it became clear even to the most ostrichlike, insensitive-to-survival city dweller that something new had come upon the scene. Violence had become mass violence, and the police openly declared they could not defend the public properly. The long-suppressed secret was out—survival was a matter of personal responsibility. The comforting notion that "they" will protect us at all times was dashed to bits. For the first time, many citizens considered buying a firearm, and for the first time, the notion of "safe areas" was being questioned. What experts and gun enthusiasts had preached for years had come true. When the chips are down, you will probably be the one who will have to protect yourself and your family. Relying on others may be too little and too late.

The color code system is obsolete for civilian use, since the conditions it functioned in have now changed. Actually, even in the military it was really only suited for warfare in a classic sense, where the battle lines were well demarcated. In guerrilla warfare, there are no such lines. The enemy is everywhere. There are no more degrees of alertness out in the jungle or in the street. There is only full alert. Civilians who step out of the properly guarded confines of their homes enter a battle zone where guerrilla warfare flourishes. Out in the street, full alert is the norm. The world of the alley cat has descended upon us all.

In Israel, terrorist crime still accounts for most injury and death. In North America, the opposite is true; standard crime is the reason. However, we are seeing an increase in both types of crimes in both areas of the globe. They are the fastest growing industries in the world; neither suffer from recession or depression.

THE SURVIVAL ALERT SYSTEM

The lessons of street survival learned in Israel have proven that the mental outlook of viewing the street at full alert is the best guarantee of surviving to a ripe old age. It is time we set the time-honored "color codes of danger" system aside. It is time for a new, less complex system. It is time for the "Survival Alert System."

Relaxed Alert: In the Home

If your home is protected by the three-circle defense system, which I have been teaching here in Israel and which I go into detail about in Chapter 8, you can be in what is called a relaxed alert. Sort of like our alley cat sunning himself on that wall.

This means your weapons are nearby, ready to be put on in an instant, and yet not in the way if you prefer to go unarmed for more comfort as you do household tasks. Firemen in North America leave their clothes and tools nearby and ready in just the same manner. They are in a state of relaxed alert, but when the bell rings they are instantly moving in a precoordinated plan as they rush from the firehouse.

Full Alert: The Street

Once I open the door of my home, I am in a state of full alert. Why? Because neither I nor anybody else can ever really know what awaits out there. I have opened my home to a battle zone.

I recently received an anxious phone call from a good

friend of mine who lives near Beverly Hills. He said eight brutal murders had occurred in a single night within a radius of only a few miles. "What's the world coming to if I can't go out for a stroll with my wife or make a deposit at a drive-in automatic teller without being murdered, and near Beverly Hills no less," he asked.

I tried to make him see that the problem is worldwide, that a woman who lives in my village was at a bus stop in broad daylight and was attacked by a criminal who tried to strangle her. A few weeks later, a taxi driver had his throat slit only 100 yards away—this only six and a half miles outside the

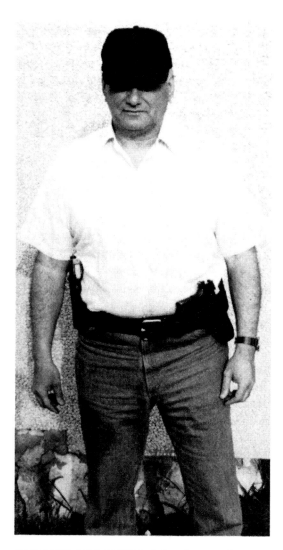

"LOADED FOR BEAR": When leaving the portals of my home, I make sure I'm well armed. A brace of matching .45 autos and plenty of ammo are considered the bare minimum.

Holy City of Jerusalem. What indeed is the world coming to? Color code systems to classify degrees of danger? Unfortunately, it's an out-of-date concept in the streets of today.

Arming for Full Alert

When I walk past the portals of my humble abode, I go "loaded for bear." The rig is the same if I'm going to feed the dogs and cats. It's the same if I'm going to work out back with my grape vines. It's the same if I am walking down the road to visit family. It's the same if I am going to a shopping mall in the city. It's the same anywhere I venture—giving lectures to Israelis on street survival, teaching a class on the shooting range, whatever. A brace of .45 autos and eight or more loaded magazines are on me. Full alert is the name of the game, and the deadly game is called survival.

Does this seem ridiculous? Paranoid? Possibly, but remember, those terrorists hit just in front of my mother's apartment. The murders that took place in Los Angeles took place in prestigious neighborhoods. The woman was attacked, the taxi driver was murdered only down the street. Recently, a young girl foolishly hitchhiking in the same area was later found raped and murdered. The street has arrived at our very doorstep.

STREET SURVIVAL LESSONS

1) *Survival alert system.* Do not think in the old manner of bad, crime-ridden neighborhoods. You can be attacked in the middle of Beverly Hills in today's world. There are no longer valid reasons to use the color code system degrees of alertness when out on the street. Danger can no longer be conveniently compartmentalized as it once was. Danger exists everywhere.

2) *Relaxed alert.* You can relax in your home if it is secure against any penetration. A relaxed state of alert has to be earned by your efforts in fortifying

your home but, once achieved, is of great comfort in an increasingly uncomfortable world.

3) *Firehouse method.* Even in a properly protected home, you should be able to react instantly to an outside danger or to someone attempting to breech your sanctuary. This means having weapons, etc., near at hand and ready. The fireman's method of readiness forms the basis of such thinking.

4) *Armed for bear.* When leaving your home, carry your weapons even if you only go out for a moment. Those serious about survival know that danger exists in the most unlikely places. Act accordingly. Comfort is nice, but survival is final.

5) *You are your own first line of defense.* Relying on others to protect you at all times is a proven formula for disaster. Top law enforcement experts admit that. The police cannot be everywhere at all times. Your alertness to danger and your ability to defend yourself and your loved ones are the only certainties you have.

SCENARIO PLANNING

It is said the late and great Herman Kahn, who headed the prestigious Hudson Institute think tank, coined the phrase "scenario planning." I have worked in two think tanks in my life, so I have grown accustomed to scenario planning as a useful tool for daily life. What we attempt to do in scenario planning is to think of a problem we may face and then work out a series of solutions to solve it, always thinking of the worst possible circumstances that may affect us (worst case scenarios). For example, say we are called to our front door by the ringing of the doorbell. How do we approach the scenario of opening the door and thus breaching the defenses we have so painstakingly constructed to keep "the beast out"? What to do? How to do it? What possibilities await us? These are the elements that go into scenario planning. Scenario planning is a prime tool of street survival. We learn survival by running through scenarios. We learn what to expect, we learn what we need to do to neutralize dangers, we learn what our mental response should be, we learn what weapons to bring into play. We sensitize our minds to an uncertain future.

If everything we do is based on scenario planning, our response to danger will become more calm. Our mind-set will move into the realm of the cool professional, away from the chaos of the rank amateur. We will have mentally experienced problems over and over again in our minds. We will have carried our carefully thought-out solutions into our tactics and training.

With scenario planning, we will become much more difficult to surprise. We will have a planned well-thought-out series of responses to a host of problems and, therefore, will have an excellent chance to correctly execute a plan that works. That is what scenario planning is all about. It's about winning.

Let us focus on a simple practical application of scenario planning and see how it operates.

Scenario: Gaining Entry to Your Home

Street predators may try to get into your home by subterfuge. You have thought out scenarios to handle this tactic. What if . . . the doorbell rings. You go to your properly locked stout door.

....

STREET SURVIVAL LESSONS

1) *Be armed.* You came to the door with a loaded pistol in hand or on your belt.

2) *Have a door peephole.* Looking through the peep-

hole, you see suspicious looking young men. You are immediately put on full alert, carrying out a preplanned scenario.

YOU: Yes?

YOUNG MAN #1: We just had an accident! Our friend needs help! He's in the car.

YOUNG MAN #2: Can we use your phone?

YOU: Tell me where the car is, I'll call for you.

STREET SURVIVAL LESSON

1) *Beware of fake emergencies.* Fake emergencies are a ploy that usually works when criminals want to gain entry into a home.

YOUNG MAN #3: Hey, Mister, you afraid? We ain't gonna bite yah.

STREET SURVIVAL LESSON

1) *Don't be shamed.* Shaming you into lowering your guard is another ploy. "Open the door and show us you're a man" is really what they are saying.

YOU: Tell me where the car is and I'll call the police for you.

STREET SURVIVAL LESSON

1) *Stick to the point.* Don't engage in conversation, don't negotiate. You will not be distracted by any attempt to shift you from your well-thought-out scenario.

[Young Man #2 looks exasperated as he turns to Young Man #1.]

YOUNG MAN #2: Bill's bleeding to death and this guy sounds like a parrot. [To you]: Let us in! He'll die!

YOUNG MAN #3: Come on, have a heart, mister. We need bandages and stuff.

STREET SURVIVAL LESSON

1) *Don't be cajoled, dissuaded, or worn down.* Yours is a fair and decent response in case the accident is for real. But you absolutely refuse to place you and your family in needless jeopardy.

YOU: I'll call the police for you. They'll be here in a minute.

STREET SURVIVAL LESSON

1) *Stick to your original offer.* The telephone call. If their friend was in such dire straits, they could have said that first and had you call. You are thinking. You stayed cool, your scenario-type thinking serving you in good stead.

YOUNG MAN #1 [smiling]: Just get the bandages, open the door, and pass them to me.

YOU [calling out to someone inside]: Harry, will you call the police?

STREET SURVIVAL LESSONS

1) *Bring matters to a head.* You have ceased conversation about the bandages. You have offered to be helpful. You are now calling the police.

2) *Make them think you are not alone.* They think that "Harry" is there, that you have a male person in the house besides you. Even if he doesn't exist, they think he does.

YOUNG MAN #3: Fuck you! Bastard! Prick! (You see them running off.)

....

This, of course, is only used as a simple example of what can happen to any of us. But by careful scenario planning, we have avoided being tricked, cajoled, shamed, insulted, or outwitted. We have been available to help someone in distress and yet have not compromised our security. Scenarios do work. The very best think tanks in the world use the technique in accessing future wars or anything of national importance. Individuals can use them, too.

BODY ALARM REACTION

Much has been written about the human body kicking into gear when the stress of combat is upon us. I am not saying this doesn't happen exactly as described by many writers, I am only suggesting there are no absolutes, and not everything fits neatly into the preconceived patterns we find in textbooks. Let us delve into what is supposed to happen, and then let's see if what we read is true for everyone all of the time.

What is Supposed to Happen

You have perceived a clear and present danger. Your brain reacts by increasing the efficiency of all systems. Your pulse speeds up, blood pressure increases, and heavy breathing occurs as the body rushes oxygen to your muscles and vital organs. This sudden massive surge of oxygen may cause what is called hyperventilation—you actually may have too much oxygen and you feel dizzy, possibly even faint. If this does not occur, one good result is your concentration has increased remarkably. You are on a oxygen high.

Next, the powerful hormone called adrenaline bursts into the body. Your vital organs and muscles are charged up with increased energy as the body awaits the supreme effort it knows it will be called upon to perform. Your hands may become cold and clammy, your face pales as blood is drained away. You may become clumsy, might even tremble, and your knees may knock. But as your strength increases, you are going to be almost immune from pain if it is inflicted on you. Your strength increases dramatically. You see your opponent through a vision process called "tunnel vision," which excludes all other objects. Your hearing also undergoes a change called "auditory exclusion" (call it tunnel vision of the ears). You may not be aware of any other dangers nor of anyone even behind your opponent. You may not be able to hear anyone shouting at you. You are hyped-up on adrenaline and oxygen, ready to "go for broke."

Is all of this possible? Most decidedly, yes. Is it the norm? Does it always happen? Can you look forward to it happening? As the song says, "It ain't necessarily so."

What is Likely to Happen

Over the years, it has been my privilege to have what I consider to be the most experienced fighters in the world as close friends or my students of shooting and survival skills. During this time, I have interviewed hundreds of Israeli combat soldiers as to their experiences in battle. Conclusion: *There are no absolutes.*

Responses seemed to fall into three broad categories.

CATEGORY #1: FIRST TIME IN COMBAT. This group was made up of soldiers who had never seen combat before. They tended to have experienced the body alarm symptoms listed above. Undoubtedly, fear of the unknown played its part in eliciting and maximizing these symptoms.

CATEGORY #2: COMBAT VETERANS. Many of these men recalled fewer signs of these body alarm reactions. They occurred sporadically and seemed to be somewhat watered down in overall effect. These men tended to be somewhat colder in their thinking about mortal combat. Combat experience helped them function much better under the stress of battle.

CATEGORY 3: "FIGHTERS." In my contact with Israeli soldiers, I tended every now and then to come across what the Israelis affectionately call a "fighter." These are men who seem born to combat, men who remind us of the heroes of the Bible—genetic throwbacks to the times of Joshua, King David, and Bar Kochba, the Jewish general who almost defeated the Roman Empire—or of American history, such as Daniel Boone, Sgt. Alvin York, Audy Murphy, and Gen. George Patton.

What astounded me about them was a lack of fear and a cold tension and determination in battle that made them seem almost calm. They were born to battle, or some say reborn. I would venture to say they almost enjoyed battle in a way that cannot be described in average terms. If they could be described in other terms, the name warrior ants comes to mind in a most respectful manner. These are the true fighters, men who seem quite at home in battle.

INTERVIEW WITH LT. COL. SCHLOMO BAUM

Many experts consider Schlomo Baum to be one of the leading experts on antiterror warfare alive today.

E.S.: The Israeli term "fighter" is often used to describe those men who excel in combat. How would you describe such a man? What attributes does he have?

S.B.: "Fighters" are men whose natural born instincts work better than the average man's, especially in battle. The first natural instinct to leave so-called civilized man is the instinct of having a sense of danger. My greatest advantage in deadly combat was my habit of looking around and seeing danger, quickly and crystal clear. Because of this ability, I was able to instantly size up the situation. I immediately knew what I had to do.

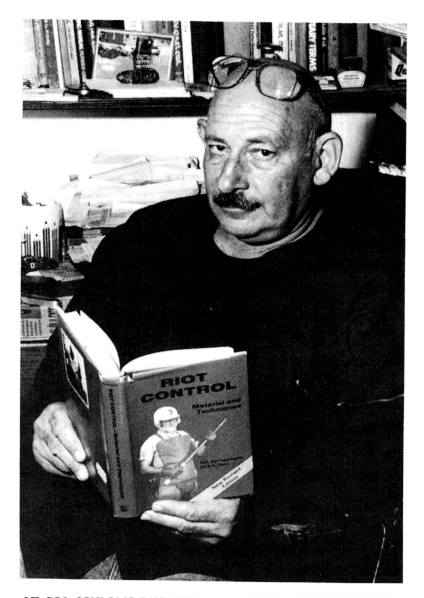

LT. COL. SCHLOMO BAUM RELAXES WITH COL. REX APPLEGATE:
Israeli expert studies U.S. expert. Baum is a relative of "The amazing Major
Baum," one of General Patton's officers who led a commando raid on a
German prisoner of war camp to free U.S. soldiers during World War II.

E.S.: This seems to call for a panoramic view of mortal combat. Isn't this diametrically opposed to so-called tunnel vision, where we tend to narrow our vision of danger, be it in the military battlefield or the civilian battlefield we call street survival?

S.B.: The phenomena of narrowed vision in combat, now labeled tunnel vision, is not new. It sometimes emerges when mortal danger is faced and is not a rare human reaction. It was during World War II that this reaction was properly described in psychiatric terms—"Tachy-Psychy effect."

I can only describe what I felt in close-quarter, be it against enemy troops or against armed terrorists on many hundreds of occasions. As I said, my greatest advantage was a coldness in battle, inbred naturally and eventually conditioned even more by battle experience. It seemed that before anyone around me even recognized the danger, I found I had already reacted to it. I call this "mastering the battlefield." Real fighters seem to have a built-in radar that responds to the most immediate threat. In other words, a keen sense of target selection that is natural to them.

E.S.: Were you born with this ability?

S.B.: Yes. When I was young and in deadly confrontations with our enemies, I had this sense of constantly looking and recognizing small details that others may not have noticed or deemed unimportant.

E.S.: Sort of like a cat?

S.B.: Cats are masters at survival, and survival is the name of the game when you are in deadly combat. Like Patton said, "I don't want you to die for your country, I want you to make the S.O.B. die for his." Incidentally, I have both dogs and cats around my house. If a stranger approaches, the cats always sense the danger faster than the dogs.

E.S.: Could you give us an example of how this sense of danger worked for you?

S.B.: It's worked for me hundreds of times, but one particular instance comes to mind. Incidentally, people like to differentiate mortal combat on the battlefield and mortal combat in "the street." This is not true. I have been in both places, and the principles of winning over your adversary are the same. Let me relate one such incident . . .

Case Study: Commando Suez Raid

Back in 1969, we were fighting the Egyptians in what was called the War of Attrition, a battle of heavy gunfire across the Suez. I pushed for an Israeli commando raid across the Gulf of Suez so that the battle would change from static warfare (which favored the Egyptians) to mobile warfare (which favored us).

We crossed the Gulf of Suez in captured Soviet armored vehicles on the night of September 8 into September 9. We could see the light coming from a place called Ras Abuderage, which was on the western shore. When we landed, our tank guns immediately opened up at an Egyptian antiaircraft and radar station. Vision was extremely poor due to the natural sand and dust in the area and to something called "les," which is a micrograined sand that whirls up at the slightest movement. Because of this, no one, the Egyptians or us, could see much of anything except the flashes from our tank guns. Prior to this, I had observed the Egyptian officers peering at us through binoculars. I felt they were confused since they saw Soviet armor (which is exactly why we used it). I was right. It took them five to eight minutes before they opened fire with Soviet 23mm quad antiaircraft guns—guns that could have shot through our Soviet APCs like a hot knife through butter.

My force [Force B] had to go down the main road, turn left, and smash through the main gate of the Egyptian fortress. I instantly visualized what I had glimpsed earlier, the whole battlefield. I knew that the Egyptians were hitting the ground about 50 meters from us, while our second force of Israeli tanks [Force A], who were facing the fort from another direction about a mile away, were not firing.

I had to make a quick decision before the heavy quads found their correct range and decimated our APC. I had ten men, 100 kilograms of high explosives, and thirty antitank mines. If hit, we would have gone up like a Roman candle.

The smoke and sand were thick now, and we couldn't see, but I pictured in my imagination what I couldn't see and decided to attack immediately. The Israeli tank commander of Force A also couldn't see, but he hesitated, didn't fire, and didn't attack. I believe he suspected the road was mined.

I knew I had to eliminate that pair of quad antiaircraft guns, so I ordered my driver to "turn left and attack!" I ordered "zig-zag," so as to make it more difficult for them to aim at us through the swirling sand, dust, and les. Again, I visualized the whole battlefield and not just a narrow area. What I didn't see I saw in my mind from what I had glimpsed before. I knew that one small error in judgment and we'd be destroyed, turning potential victory into a horrible disaster.

As we charged forward, my second in command shouted, "Schlomo [Solomon in English], no one is following us!"

"Charge!" I yelled, knowing that we had to crush the enemy by ourselves or perish.

As we moved down a narrow road we came upon something I had glimpsed before and had burned into my mind. The enemy had wedged a truck piled high with barrels filled with burning diesel fuel in between a 3-meters-deep-and-wide ridge that the road passed through. We had to get through it without spilling the blazing diesel fuel over our high explosives. All this while the antiaircraft quads spewed their deadly bullets just over our heads.

The heat from the burning diesel was intense. I ordered the medic to wet a towel in water to cover my head as I ordered my driver, who was seated below me, to slowly push the blazing truck back. My driver was cool and courageous, repeating each of my commands as I stared up at the burning barrels high above my head, watching them shake as the truck was pushed back inch by inch. Vision was good since our APC was of a roofless, open design. What was bad about all of this was the distinct possibility that a barrel of burning diesel fuel could splash down over all of us.

My driver slowly pushed the blazing enemy truck up the road at a steep angle. Near the end I caught a glimpse of the enemy fortress through the sand and smoke as we pushed the truck off of a 100-meter-high cliff, tossing it blazing into the sea.

The enemy were dumbfounded at our audacity and actually stopped firing for about 30 seconds, enough time for us to charge and overwhelm them and thus secure victory. I have seen it before in mortal combat—audacity sometimes overwhelms your enemy and gives you a slight advantage, which you should capitalize on by pressing forward the attack with all of your power.

I quizzed Baum on what lessons of street survival he could draw from that military battle:

··

STREET SURVIVAL LESSONS

1) *You control the fight.* Never let your enemy control and fight the kind of battle they would like to fight. Turn the tables on him and fight the kind of fight you want.

2) *Surprise is everything.* Use it to win unevenly matched battles where you are seemingly at a disadvantage. This was done by the Israelites of the Bible when they faced much stronger odds. It works today.

3) A *ferocious counterattack,* especially when coupled with surprise, is the best way to throw your enemy off balance and win. Attack, attack, and then attack again. Never give up.

4) *Have a mental picture of the battle zone.* Poor visibility means you have to burn a fleeting picture of the immediate environment into your mind. For example, a pistol shoot-out in the darkness of the night—learn to do this fast.

5) *Never give up.* Never accept even the idea of defeat. Think only of victory and act accordingly. Do this in a most decisive manner. Think

win. Fight to win. Use boldness and audacity to your advantage.

....

FIGHT, FLIGHT, OR FREEZE?

All living creatures, when faced with danger, have two choices: to fight or to run away (flight). I have added a third choice—to just freeze. This occurs most vividly when a rabbit is faced by a deadly snake. Result: one well-fed snake.

Freezing

This phenomenon occurs when an individual faced with danger finds he or she cannot even run. It is a severe form of fright and is not uncommon. Of the three choices, freezing is the most dangerous. In human beings it may be brought about by an utter lack of the ability to face even the idea of danger. These are usually the individuals who live by the mottos, "I couldn't live that way," "I don't want to hurt anyone," or "I would rather die than kill."

These poor souls have never made any scenario plans in their minds, deeming them too painful and horrible to even consider. Many of these individuals are against firearms of any kind and fear them along with anything else even remotely related to self-defense. They are usually more capable of feeling sorry for the vicious murderers they read about in newspapers or see on TV than for their helpless victims.

They believe in a most cowardly manner that appeasement of evil can stop evil. They are like dogs who roll over in a subservient position when faced with the presence of a more dominant dog. Incidentally, in nature, the dominant dog usually accepts their submission. This is not true in the human context, the nature of criminals being that anyone in the freezing position excites and enrages them, stimulating them to mayhem and murder.

Avoid the "freezers" like the plague. They are born victims.

Flight

The ability to retreat and fight another day is not an unrealistic thing to do when faced with overwhelming odds. Even the most aggressive commanders in military history have sometimes been forced to use flight. The Battle of Dunkerque is a classic example of when the tactic of flight saved an entire army (the British Expeditionary Force) to fight another day.

In my opinion, flight should be done only if it does not put innocents at risk. However, if you are sufficiently armed and innocents are put at risk by your flight, then flight under these circumstances is dishonorable.

Case Study: The Maalot Massacre

One evening, an Israeli school bus stopped at a religious school at Nat, a northern Israeli town located close to the Lebanese border. One hundred children and their male teachers on a school outing disembarked and entered the building to sleep there for the night.

Later that evening, six terrorists entered the building with the plan of kidnapping the children and holding them hostage for the release of hundreds of terrorists held in Israeli prisons.

At the first sign of entry, the teachers jumped out the windows and ran away, leaving the children behind. Within minutes, the authorities were alerted to what had happened. For the next 14 hours, the Israelis negotiated with the terrorists, who spoke to them through loudspeakers.

The situation rapidly deteriorated, and the Israelis, seeing that the massacre of the children was imminent, had elements of their special elite unit Syeret Mat-kal, the Chief of Staff's Scouts, storm the building and kill the terrorists.

Twenty-two children were found dead, with many more wounded, most of them seriously. One special forces Israeli commando died in the close-quarter shoot-out.

I use this unfortunate incident as a horrible example of where flight can be a most cowardly act. The teachers said they had left their issued weapons (Uzis) on the bus. They were therefore unarmed. However, they did not jump from the school windows to obtain their weapons. They fled for their lives. Innocent children left in their charge were abandoned to the terrorists. No attempt was made by the teachers to help them in any way.

....

STREET SURVIVAL LESSONS

1) *Know your weapon.* When you carry a weapon, be sure to know how to use it. The teachers were not proficient in the use of their Uzis and, under stress, fear took over since the weapons offered them no feelings of comfort or security.

2) *Always have weapons near at hand.* Always have your weapons near enough at hand so that you can reach them in a dire emergency. The teachers left their weapons on the bus in a clear violation of common sense and standing orders. However, we must offer one thing in their defense. Once again we must stress that, like all untrained people who are issued weapons, they were afraid of them and thought they and the children were safer without them.

3) *Do not believe in best-case scenarios.* Don't live in a world of fantasy. The teachers did not believe that evil could befall them, since the terrorists were across the border and the border was guarded. Lacking any worst-case-scenario plan and being totally untrained to handle such a situation, they chose flight and everlasting condemnation as despicable cowards who abandoned children to their cruel fate. It was reported at the time that the teachers left the country, fearing retribution by an irate Israeli public. (NOTE: It was said the terrorists all had their heads ventilated by the Israeli

SWAT team that stormed the building. Not one terrorist survived.)

Today, Israeli teachers undergo weapons training and some exposure to scenario thinking. They are armed. They are conditioned not to use flight as a means of facing reality.

On a regular basis, the Ministry of Education brings in experts to inspect the status of the training and make suggestions. I served as one of these outside experts a few years back. I saw the difficulties of turning teachers into security personnel. The task is a formidable one, but there is no doubt the arming and training of teachers to blunt terrorist attacks has improved the situation since the time of the tragic Maalot Massacre.

Fight

Fight is when we turn the tables on our criminal tormentors and make life hell for them. This means outgunning the gunman. Facing down a mob bent on blood. Terrorizing the terrorist. It means turning the tables on your adversary and, by the correct mind-set, tactics, and training, grinding him into the ground in a most certain and devastating manner.

Fight is also part of what is called deterrent strategy. When it is known that an individual (or a nation) makes shedding of its blood cost dearly, deterrence reaches its highest level. Fight saves lives in the long run because it gives evil pause.

Determination Wins over Muscle

Probably the best example in nature of the power of fight is in a small animal that inhabits the woods of North America. It hovers only inches above the ground and marks its territory by urinating on the trees in a wide circle. When the huge grizzly meanders up to the circle, it stops dead in its tracks, sniffs, turns around, then runs like hell. I've suggested that Israel import this creature and make it a national symbol. It's called the Wolverine. It's the real king of the woods since even a grizzly bear, weighing hundreds of pounds more and standing many feet above it, doesn't relish meeting and engaging it in a fight even when the odds are seemingly in the bear's favor. You see, the grizzly can beat the wolverine in battle, but at the price of one or two of his feet, which that little bundle of sheer fight will chew off as it dies. Grizzlies aren't that stupid; they want no part of such fighters and go off for easier pickings. In this case, the determination to fight stops aggression and saves blood from being spilled needlessly. A good model for street survival.

CORRECT MIND-SET CONQUERS ALL

Earlier in this chapter, I spoke of those individuals who are born "fighters." They almost instinctively know what to do when faced with deadly force. They do not all look like Rambo of Hollywood fame and fantasy. I have observed many of these men over the years, and while most are athletic and strong, this is not always the case. Just as with villains, the good guys, the heroes, don't always look the part.

I once asked a good friend of mine (now gone to his Maker), Paratroop Lt. Col. Hanon Davidson, about this. He told me not every man who looks like he is a fighter is capable of doing the courageous thing. Many times he observed big talkers and braggarts simply fall to pieces when confronted with the reality of deadly combat. He had also observed men who were the last people you would think of as fighters rise to the occasion when suddenly faced with mortal danger. During the cease-fire in the 1973 Yom Kippur War between Israel and Egypt, he told me an illustrative story of how a so-called nonfighter rose to the task in battle and fooled all and sundry with his innate bravery.

Case Study: The Railway Station Battle
The tide of battle in the Yom Kippur War turned when Gen. Arik Sharon sent a crack, battle-hardened paratroop brigade across the Suez Canal to secure the Egyptian shore

for movement of Israeli armor across the canal from Sinai into Egypt so as to cut off the Egyptian 3rd Army. Hanon led the first rubber dingy across the canal, and they moved into Egypt. Within a short time they were taking casualties. Paratroopers were dropping all around him. It was pitch dark, and they could not see the enemy, yet the enemy was firing one shot at a time and killing his buddies. (The Israelis did not know at the time that the Soviets had equipped the Egyptian Commandos with SLS night equipment.) Sensing that they were in a no-win situation, Hanon ordered his paratroopers into abandoned enemy bunkers, grabbed a field radio, and called for an artillery strike. At first, the Israeli artillery battery across the canal in Sinai refused, saying that their maps clearly showed that the paratroopers were in the zone to be shelled. Hanon, who was not above telling tall tales, calmly lied and told them the map was wrong. They believed his ruse, and suddenly, the earth shook as shell after shell slammed into their zone. It went on all night. When the sun came up, the Israeli paratroopers crawled out of the Egyptian bunkers to find dozens and dozens of enemy commandos blown to bits by the heavy shelling. Parts of SLS scopes were strewn over the bloody battlefield.

Once the beachhead was secured, Hanon led a trio of old white personnel-carrier half-tracks deep into Egypt and outraced the brigade. He drove into a railway junction that contained thousands of Egyptians. A heavy firefight ensued, and the Israelis were soon running out of ammunition. Suddenly, a Palestinian Arab (from a unit attached to the Egyptians) charged toward the APC, yelling and firing his SKS. Hanon was struck in the jaw and lost a few teeth. Pulling his trusty Colt 1911 (we had trained together—this was the pistol I had recommended to him), he let the PLO guy have a 230-grain jacketed ball square in his chest. The attacker fell back like a felled tree. At this, the APCs turned around and fought their way out of the area.

Hanon fell back, bleeding to death. It was here that the unexpected happened. A little driver called Hamoodee ("darling" in Hebrew), whose parents had immigrated to Israel from the Yemen, grabbed some maps and forced them into Hanon's wound to stem the bleeding. This he did as he drove the APC and fired his weapon. The unit battled its way back to the Israeli lines. When they got to a field hospital, Hanon was thrown on an operating table. Up to the time of the surgery, Hamoodee held those maps in the wound, stemming the flow of blood. Hanon lived to fight another day, saved by his driver who demonstrated courage and a never-say-die fighting spirit.

Hanon mused that Hamoodee was a most unlikely hero; he just didn't look the part. Yet when faced with danger, he rose to the occasion and persevered. Where other men may have panicked, the little guy did three jobs at once under a deadly hail of enemy fire and succeeded in doing all of them quite well.

(Oh, incidentally, Israeli field security came into the operating room, spotted those secret maps that Hamoodee had used, and chewed him out for bringing them back from the front line. Pencil-pushing bureaucrats, the same the world over.)

....

STREET SURVIVAL LESSONS

1) *Never say die.* Though seriously wounded, Hanon didn't quit. He pulled his .45 auto and dispatched his attacker with one well-placed shot right before he collapsed.

2) *Correct mind-set.* Hamoodee proved you don't have to physically look like a fighter to be one. The will to fight is what really counts.

3) *Backup weapon.* That .45 auto saved Hanon's life since his M1 Carbine (he liked that weapon) was out of ammo.

SURVIVAL INSTINCT

The instinct to survive seems basic to all living organisms. Nature was created in a system of checks and balances—life lives on life and the fittest survive. In many creatures, the instinct to survive encompasses the adult's instinct for protecting the young and the weak of the species. It is all a natural development of the instinct of protecting one's own from danger.

If this instinct for survival is so basic to life itself, how can we explain some of our fellow human beings who seem bent on committing suicide by not looking evil in the face and taking the steps necessary to defeat it? What has happened to their basic sense of survival? How has this happened to our species?

Unfortunately, there are some people who roam the earth who do not have the survival instinct of the common housefly or mosquito. Move toward one of these tiny creatures with fly swatter in hand and they fly away. They feel danger approaching. Mosquitoes even seem to sense when someone is staring at them. On the other hand, there are some people who simply refuse to face reality, suppressing the instinct for survival and replacing it with a false creed, a creed based on the mistaken assumption that if you treat people nicely, they will reciprocate in kind. No more basic and dangerous error in survival could be made. Such a false creed goes against the very laws of nature and almost ensures that sooner or later the price will be paid.

Case Study: Bloody Murder at Bar Ilad

NOTE: The details and names in this (and other cases) have been changed so as to protect the living—in this case from the pain of reliving its tragic consequences.

Bar Ilad is a famous tourist attraction in the north of the State of Israel that contains some of the most wonderful natural springs in the world. It is open from 9 A.M. to 9 P.M., run by a very dedicated man named Amos. Now Amos was a very special sort of person who was incapable of inflicting any pain on any fellow human being and assumed that others felt the same way about him. His philosophy led him to be friends with two guys who worked nearby, and they spent many an hour together drinking the strong, sweet Turkish coffee that is so popular in this part of the world and which greases the wheels of good fellowship.

One day Amos came to work at 7 A.M. to do some office work. He left the door to his office open, since he believed a locked

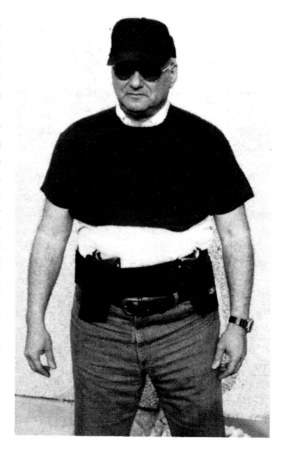

BACKUP WEAPON: Always carry a backup weapon. This is true even when you have a long gun as a primary weapon.

door insulted his good friends, who would look upon such an act as a very unfriendly thing to do. Amos also didn't carry a firearm for the same reason. He believed, like many, that guns invite trouble.

It was 9 A.M. when his body was found. He had more than 100 stab wounds on his body. The doctor who examined him said they were inflicted in a frenzy of murderous thrusts. Within days his two good friends were arrested and readily confessed to the murder. When asked why they chose to kill him that day, they replied, "We were walking by and saw the door open. We knew Amos never carried a gun or any other form of protection. We pulled our knives and stabbed him. We didn't hate Amos, in fact we liked him very much, but you see, he was an Israeli and we are Arabs. What else could we have done?"

STREET SURVIVAL LESSONS

1) *Fear of danger helps you survive.* Amos' natural-born instinct for survival was suppressed and watered down by an unnatural philosophy that made him not only more vulnerable to attack, but actually helped to invite it.

2) *Common sense is critical.* Common sense is a basic survival tool. Common sense should have warned Amos that he was in danger. But, as Schlomo Baum likes to say, "Eugene, one thing I've learned: common sense . . . is not so common."

Case Study: Stabbing at Erez

Erez is an industrial zone just across the so-called Green Line (the 1967 border) from Gaza. An Israeli businessman named Meir Asour, 35, and other members of his family have a warehouse there.

At about 7 A.M., Asour felt a blow to his back. (Many times a knife stab doesn't hurt, being perceived as a fist.) He spun around and saw that Tamer Zeyara, 17, who had been a trusted Arab worker at Asour's family clothing business for about two years, was pointing a long knife at his chest. Asour instinctively tried to ward off the second blow with his open hand and lost one of his fingers in the process as his hand was split almost in half.

"I turned around and drew my handgun with difficulty,"

said Asour, "because I had been stabbed in the hand . . . and shot him in the head a few times [early reports claimed five]. Then I collapsed." The press reported that Zeyara's uncle, Bakar, said, "My nephew belonged to Hamas and wanted to die as a martyr. He did die as a martyr, and I am proud of him."

A note was found in Tamer Zeyara's pocket saying he had received money (less than $200) from the fundamentalist Islamic Jihad to murder an Israeli.

Members of the Asour family expressed astonishment that Tamer Zeyara had attempted to murder Meir Asour, who they said had always treated Tamer with kindness and respect. They just can't believe that their friend and trusted worker could have been a member of the fanatical Hamas organization.

STREET SURVIVAL LESSONS

1) *Never lower your guard.* Jonathan claims that in the United States, most officers of the law who are killed while on duty are murdered by people out there in the street whom they know. Familiarity tends to lower one's survival instinct. Tamer Zeyara used his relationship with Meir Asour to get close to and behind him. He almost succeeded in his murder attempt.

2) *Avoid Condition #3 carry.* Asour made a second mistake, that of carrying his auto pistol in Condition #3, empty chamber. He had to pull back the slide to load his weapon—all this while holding off a knife-wielding attacker and after his hand had been sliced almost in half.

3) *Careful of gun oil.* Asour made a third mistake. He had sprayed a highly penetrative oil into his gun and had deactivated his first round when the oil leaked into it. He had to pull back the slide again after he suffered a misfire.

4)　*At close quarters, aim for the head.* While head zone shots against a moving target at a range of more than a few yards are extremely difficult and are not recommended, when right up against your attacker, shoot for the head if you can. What Meir Asour did superbly well was to drive those bullets into Zeyara's head, and he kept firing until Zeyara was dead. If he had not done this, chances are that when Asour collapsed he may have been stabbed again, almost certainly with fatal results.

5)　*First priority—your back.* Never let anyone get behind you whom you don't totally trust. Even then, remember that alley cat. You should experience some uneasiness when someone goes behind you. It's a healthy feeling that shows you are cautious.

OVERCOMING CULTURAL CONDITIONING

We live under an umbrella of a Western culture that teaches us restraint in the face of violence. This is not true of other cultures of the world, nor is it even true in some of the subcultures that flourish under that umbrella. Those of us who have been taught from birth that turning the other cheek is laudable or have heard the cliché "nice boys don't fight" are at a distinct psychological disadvantage when facing those who have been taught the opposite from birth. To survive in the street against such predators, we must overcome cultural conditioning. It's not a simple task to rethink what has been inculcated into us from our first breath on this earth. I challenge the very idea that to turn the other cheek is somehow an act of holiness. It is exactly the opposite.

Mistranslation of the Second Biblical Commandment
The Bible forms the basis of our cultural conditioning.

Few laymen know that the Second Commandment was mistranslated from the original Hebrew into Greek, and then into English. Almost daily, we hear the words, "Thou shalt not kill." This has been expanded from the killing of man to include deer, foxes, rabbits, mice, etc. It has been used as one of the basic tenants of the vegetarian movement, and for the antihunting lobby's sanctimonious, quasimoralistic preachings. *The Bible does not say this.*

The original Hebrew reads, "Thou shalt not murder." In other words, you are not to shed the blood of your innocent fellow human beings in vain. It certainly has nothing to do with animals. The Bible further clarifies the matter and reads, "If someone comes to kill you, get up and kill him first." Therefore, self-defense is not only justified, it is a direct order from the Almighty! Hmmm . . . doesn't that begin to give you a new perspective on life?

The Bible further states (to paraphrase), "He who has pity on the merciless has no mercy on the pitiful." Meaning: if you take pity on evil, you doom the innocent, the weak, and the good. As the Englishman Edmund Burke wrote, "The only thing necessary for the triumph of evil is for good men to do nothing."

I have never ceased to marvel at how many other Biblical mistranslations from the original Hebrew are bantered about every day by those who should know better. These monumental and critical errors have had a profound effect on all kinds of movements around the world. However, the mistranslation of the second Biblical commandment is probably the most deadly one. It has caused the death of many people who thought it holy not to resist evil.

It would be comical if so many human beings had not actually thrown their lives away in pursuit of the false precept that to capitulate to evil is somehow holy. It is not. The most holy book known to Western civilization, in its original Hebrew, says the exact opposite. Self-defense against evil is holy. Something to ponder when attempting to achieve the correct mind-set for street survival.

STREET SURVIVAL LESSON

1)   *Attack evil.* Don't feel guilty about defending yourself from evil attack. The Bible actually commands you to do so. It is considered a just deed. The only way to protect the weak and innocent is by destroying evil.

Can You Learn to Be a Fighter?

We now know that some people are born to battle, just as some are born to music, basketball, or creative writing. But we also know that these things can be learned and within the physical and mental limitations of each individual. Some of us, with practice and determination, can accomplish these tasks when called upon to do so. How can we go about becoming "fighters" who can survive in the streets when facing deadly force? We do know that even individuals who have shown cowardice under fire and survived have sometimes undergone a metamorphosis and turned into deadly adversaries the next time around. Is there a method, some way, some key, by which each of us can improve our street survival capabilities? The answer is an emphatic *yes.*

THREE LEVELS OF STREET SURVIVAL

Level #1: The Conscious Level

This is the level of the novice (for our purposes, we hope the novice comes to us with strong motivation brought about by a keen realization that shooting trophies and medals, while fun to win, have absolutely no relationship to deadly combat).

Beginning the learning process at this level is what is called the conscious level. Here the person learning street survival tactics and weaponry is relying 100 percent on his conscious perception of what he is doing.

At this level a technique is introduced, talked about,

thought about, and deliberately executed. The whole idea seems rough in execution; nothing moves smoothly. It's very much like what the amateur does rather than the professional. Conditioned reflexes are just about nonexistent. It's all thought out.

In the military, it's the time of the raw recruit. In the police, it's the time of the police academy. For the individual, it could be the first time on the shooting range. This is not to say that seasoned fighters don't go through this phase every time they learn something new; they do. However, experience makes the process pass by faster, with seemingly less effort.

Even Truck Drivers Die

I've trained students who ranged from novice to elite commando. Believe me, it's easier to train elite commandos. I remember one afternoon I spent among many hundreds in my paratroop unit, the one Hanon belonged to. We were on the shooting range, zeroing in our new M16 rifles that had just been flown into Israel in Galaxy cargo planes, an emergency airlift from the States. This was during the cease-fire of the Yom Kippur war of 1973.

A group of soldiers showed up with their rifles, and I noticed that their boots were black and not the brownish red ones Israeli paratroopers wore. However, I thought they belonged to the Brigade, so I proceeded to help them zero their weapons. After a few hours of range work I was coming to the conclusion that either I was having a particularly bad day or these were a particularly slow bunch of learners. Suddenly, a jeep pulled up and an officer jumped out and pulled me aside, asking, "Why are you spending so much time with these truck drivers? They just bring us supplies, they're not 'fighters.'"

I turned to see them looking anxiously in my direction. I said to the officer, "Do they have an agreement with the Syrians that they won't be fired at?" The officer looked at me in surprise, smiled, and confessed to me they hadn't such an agreement. He jumped back into his jeep and drove away.

I spent the rest of the afternoon with those truck drivers

and can inform you that each of them hugged me a thankful good-bye when they left, saying, "Thanks for helping us upgrade our chances of surviving." (Come to think of it, one of the nicest things ever said to me.)

Level #2: The Subconscious Level

The ideal in street survival is having what you learned at the conscious Level #1 become second nature to you, the so-called conditioned reflex Level #2. This is the level where you respond automatically to a threat, doing what you are trained to without having to think about it.

One of the criticisms I and many others have about so-called practical pistol shooting as it's done today is that it has turned into a sport which has little, if any, relationship to self-defense. It could even be argued that the opposite is true in that many of the techniques and exercises stressed are actually dangerous to one's street survival. I am not only speaking about outlandish pistols with laser sights held in totally impractical street rigs. That we could at least live with. I am speaking about an exercise that fires a double tap (two quick bullets in succession) at an adversary, then moves on and repeats the same double tap to each target down the shooting line. This is a surefire formula for getting killed out in the street, where the third adversary won't be waiting like a dead paper target for you to get to him. I preached against the El Presidente exercise way back in the early 1960s. I still haven't changed my mind.

Most shooters I spoke to claimed that they understood it was wrong, but they only did it when they were at their local practical pistol shooting club and swore they would never do such a stupid thing when faced with an armed street gang who decided to partake of their wallet or their wife. My stock answer has always been, "You are what you eat. You are what you practice. When the chips are down I (and any psychiatrist worth his salt) promise you, you will do exactly as you practiced, no more and no less." When training Israeli Commando Scouts, I used to stress this point over and over.

Incidentally, the correct thing to do when using lethal firearm force against a group of adversaries is to engage each one with a single bullet, going up the line and then double tapping the last one in line, then repeating the single shot to each one as you come back. Of course, such a pat sequence is unlikely, but we must practice the basic principles on the shooting range so that we engage close-quarter targets, all of them, as quickly and decisively as possible. If we are foolish enough to double tap each one, it is almost guaranteed that adversary #3 will finish you.

In honing our skills to reach Level #2, we must understand the principles of what we are trying to learn as well as the actual mechanics of achieving said goal. Learning the correct way is just as easy as learning the incorrect way, but the results out there in the street are decisive either way.

We must keep in mind that although Level #2 culminates in our reaching our goal of doing what we trained for in a subconscious way, it is not totally subconscious in execution—not yet. Why? Because we are still focusing on each of many thoughts in the sequence needed for correct performance. We are concentrating too much rather then flowing with the action. An example would be concentrating on blinking our eyes correctly when an object is thrown at us rather then doing it automatically and without concentration as we do instinctively. We want to achieve the ultimate goal of Level #3, for example, the convulsive grip and the crouch we all assume naturally, without thinking, when hot lead starts to fly.

Level #3: The Israeli Fighter's Level

This is the supreme level of combat, the level of "fighters." It is possible to learn Level #3 through proper mind-set and training. The ideal is allowing our conscious mind to handle what it does best, figuring out what to do in a lethal confrontation, while our subconscious mind takes care of the actual mechanics of weapon control, etc. To achieve this, repetitious, correct training is necessary so that every self-defense skill is on autopilot. Like the good Colonel Baum, you are now totally aware of everything in your immediate environment, and nothing distracts you from street survival.

You are not thinking about how to place your front sight on target or which artery to cut in your adversary's body. You have finally become a fighting machine, one very difficult for some scumbag to cut down in the street.

Level #3 is the ultimate goal. It can be achieved with constant, diligent, correct practice with whatever weapons you choose. It can be achieved mentally—the correct mind-set—so that you have all possible scenarios stored away in your subconscious mind ready for instant use.

STREET SURVIVAL LESSONS

1) *You are what you practice.* Never practice, partake, or compete in shooting games (or any combat-oriented games) that teach anything that is against the basic rules and skills needed for street survival.

2) *You can learn to be a "fighter."* If you do not feel like a born "fighter" do not give up hope. With perseverance, you can learn to become one by using the time-proven Three-Level System of training.

3) *Everyone can learn street survival.* Never give up hope when you want someone (your wife?) to learn how to defend themselves. Those Israeli truck drivers didn't lack guts, they just lacked technique. Once someone wants to learn, you're 90-percent there. First, motivate them, and then the rest is easy. Never give up on anyone, and that includes yourself.

THE LAW AND YOU

Never be ignorant of the law. Ignorance in this case is not

bliss. Taking the life of a fellow human being is a very final act. The decision must be well thought out. You must have a firm idea where you stand legally, since the legal consequences and ramifications of such an action can be quite intimidating and can hurt you in two ways. First, using deadly force when it is not indicated can get you in a pack of trouble, including a murder charge. Conversely, not using deadly force when it is indicated can win you a quick trip to the undertaker.

This book cannot be used to form a legal opinion to base any decision on the use of deadly force. Only the knowledge of the laws governing deadly force in your jurisdiction can do that. Remember, these laws may be different where you live. They can be subject to change. So forewarned is fore-armed. Beware. Check the laws carefully. In the street, ignorance of the law breeds hesitation; hesitation can kill.

DEADLY FORCE

This legal term is a catch-all phrase that simply means the

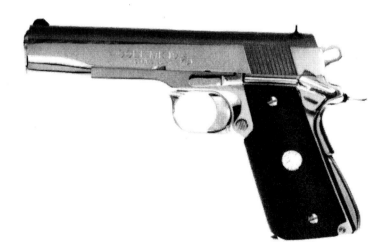

COLT SERIES 80 MK IV: A good, solid modern 1911 with a firing pin safety that almost ruins it. Some of the triggers on these pistols are not exactly a joy to use.

manner you use—firearm, knife, club, hammer, your bare hands, etc.—to kill an assailant.

Common Law

This refers to what is called English common law, the unwritten law that forms the basis of much of what passes for law in the English-speaking world. Under common law, deadly force cannot be used if all you want to do is protect property. An unarmed burglar would not be considered a prime candidate for deadly force. However, if said burglar has a deadly weapon, such as a firearm or a knife, and makes a threatening move, and you have a reasonable fear for your life or that of your family, common law allows you to use deadly force.

Reasonable Fear

This term is the key to the puzzle of the use of deadly force. The problem is, how can you prove violent intent of the burglar if you don't allow him to make the first move and thus place you and your family at risk? Unfortunately, no one has ever come up with a really clear answer. The law is therefore weighted on the side of the criminal. Unfair? You bet it is. That's why you must have scenarios worked out in your mind regarding when to use deadly force. Even then you still could face judge and jury.

Immediate Danger

The courts believe that this is a very important factor in whether your use of deadly force was justified. The street punk facing you outside a bar cannot be engaged with lethal weapons if he says, "I'm goin' home and get my gun, then I'm comin' back and I'm gonna blow your brains out." Why? Because the danger is not immediate. He did not pull a gun and say, "Motherfucker, I'm gonna shoot you!" When this occurs, the danger you face is immediate, and you have no choice if you want to live. In this case lethal force is justified.

Is the Danger Unavoidable?

Let's say you go down the street toward a street punk who has sworn to kick your butt or worse. You see him. He did not see you. You say to yourself, "Screw him. I have a gun in my pocket waiting for that bastard to carry out his threat." You walk up to him and, lo and behold, he reacts just as he said he would and you ventilate his guts with three .45-caliber hollowpoints, killing him in the process. Don't be surprised if the court verdict rules you guilty because the situation was avoidable.

Deadly Danger

If that street punk kicks you in your private parts while he insists you are guilty of incest, shooting him is still deemed unjustified. Unless the danger is that as a reasonable and prudent person you would deem him liable to cause death or grievous bodily harm (not momentary pain), resulting in your being crippled, you are in deep feces for using your deadly weapon.

Killing the Innocent

Let's say you are at home watching a football game, and five men smash down your front door and storm in brandishing shotguns and wearing raid jackets with the letters POLICE written across them. You jump up and empty your revolver at them; one dies. You, kind sir, are in deep trouble. Why? You should have known that anyone wearing such a jacket was probably a police officer who made an error and kicked the wrong door in. Cops in the United States, for example, don't go around kicking in doors and scaring honest citizens with shotguns. You don't know that? Well, that means you are not a prudent and reasonable person as far as the courts are concerned and must be punished. You were expected to offer no resistance and should have sat down with the officers and reasoned with them. That's the law. Is it all unfair? Probably; however, with street crime growing by leaps and bounds around the world, it pays for all of us to take such scenarios into consideration. Worst-case-scenario planning helps us be more prudent and reasonable.

Are You Authorized to Protect Someone?

Assuming things without knowing them for sure is one sure way to have the law against you. In many parts of the world, you are only allowed to use deadly force in defense of yourself, family, servants, and maybe workers and customers in your establishment.

That is all. No one else. That includes that woman being raped in the middle of main street by some maniac—shoot him and you may be in lots of legal trouble. You may not be authorized to protect that poor damsel in distress. Look up the laws where you live and find out what they say about deadly force. You may be very surprised.

Case Study: Damned If You Do, Damned If You Don't

Eddie Griven lives near the biblical city of Hebron in southern Israel, a place called Kiryat Arba. He came to the country in the 1950s, after he served in the U.S. armed forces during the "police action" called the Korean War. I interviewed him.

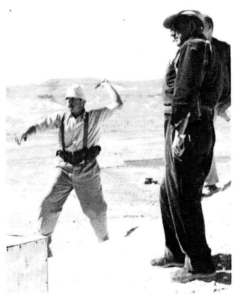

EDDIE: Teaching the boys how to throw.

E.S.: You said the law can sometimes be murky about when and how a civilian can use deadly force in coming to the aid of someone under attack.

E.G.: Heck, yeah. I was sitting on my bed reading one day when my neighbor who was in the civil guard stormed in and yelled that some guy was raping a woman in the next building. He seemed quite unprepared about how to handle the situation.

E.S.: What did you do?

E.G.: I grabbed my Colt 1911 and ran to the next building.

E.S.: What did you find?

E.G.: Exactly what he said. Some guy had his pants down and was in the process of attempting to rape a housewife. I challenged the perpetrator to cease and desist.

E.S.: Did he?

E.G.: Hell, no. He charged at me, a big guy, cursing and all. I let him have three .45 slugs square in his private parts and he stopped in his tracks.

E.S.: You must have been a hero.

E.G.: Well, now. That depends.

E.S.: Depends?

E.G.: Yeah. Depends. The Israeli army wanted to give me a medal. The problem was the Israeli police wanted to put me in jail.

E.S.: What finally happened?

E.G.: They compromised. I didn't get the medal, and I didn't go to jail.

E.S.: Would you do it again?

E.G.: Hell, yeah. Oh, incidentally, I paid a visit to the hospital where the guy I shot was.

E.S.: You wanted to speak to him?

E.G.: Hell, no. I wanted to check the X rays to see how those .45 jacketed ball slugs tracked. Funny thing happened. The rapist saw me walk by his room and he went nuts. He ran down the hall, tubes, bottles, and plastic bags dragging behind. He was yelling that I had come to finish him off. He was an Arab, you see, and in his culture that's what he would have done. Me, I was only going to check out those .45 slugs. Incidentally, they worked real well.

E.S.: What happened to the rapist?

E.G.: He went to prison. I saw him years later after he was released. He used two canes to get around, used to sit out on his front porch with his brothers when my sons and I walked past on the way to pray at the Cave of Machpela where Abraham and his family are buried.

E.S.: Have any second thoughts? Regrets?

E.G.: Hell, yeah. Should have shot the bastard in the chest.

The Assailant

The right to use lethal force against an assailant could be determined by three very critical factors: ability, opportunity, and jeopardy.

Ability

This is when your assailant possesses the means to kill or cripple. This usually means some weapon of death, though in the United States it could mean so-called "disparity of force."

Disparity of force is when your assailant is unarmed with any conventional weapon but that the sheer size and strength he possesses in and of themselves, in combination with his criminal intent, become a deadly danger.

Some examples where the doctrine of disparity of force may possibly apply are as follows:

a)   You are outnumbered by a gang of street punks bent on pounding you into the ground.

b)   You are a petite female who is attacked by a male assailant who has far superior strength.

c)   You are up against a known expert in martial arts, professional boxing, wrestling, etc., which makes his skill a lethal weapon.

d)   You are small in stature and strength and face
        another human being who far outclasses you in
        size and strength and who has violent intentions.
        The problem is, no one has ever charted what size
        or strength is considered to outclass the potential
        victim so that he may use deadly force to stop an
        attack. This is the most "dicey" of all examples.

e)   You are physically disabled and face an assailant
        who is physically capable. Maybe you are in a leg
        cast and can't run away. Possibly you are in a
        wheelchair. Or, your assailant is young and strong
        while you are far "over the hill." Once again, be
        forewarned—the courts are very subjective in
        their interpretations of what is justified. The
        attacker must be very vicious and cruel in his
        manner and method. It can't just be a big loud-
        mouthed bully who swears at you and is pushing
        you around.

Opportunity

Let's say the four gang members you face have the power
to kill or maim you, but are presently incapable of carrying
out the deed. For example, the potential assailants are yelling
at you from behind a closed door. They may be unarmed; you
don't even know. If you order them to leave and they refuse,
you may not shoot. However, if they break the door down
and charge at you, you can. It is a well-known fact that the
average person bent on mayhem can run 8 yards in about 1.5
seconds and do you in. This has been the case here in Israel
when terrorists armed with bladed weapons charged individuals armed with firearms and succeeded in stabbing them.

Jeopardy

Your attacker must be acting in such a manner that our
reasonable and prudent potential victim would assume his
intent to murder or cripple him. How can you measure such
a thing so that a court is satisfied? The answer, of course, is

you can't. Could he have been only kidding? Were you imag-
ining his bad body language, evil look, tone of voice, or even
body cue that he was about to attack? Who knows? Not even
the Shadow does.

Retreat?
Let's say your attacker has clearly displayed his ability to

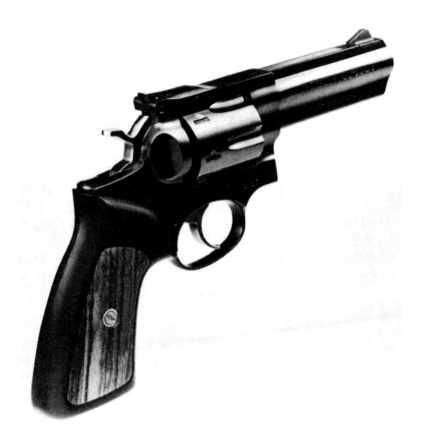

*RUGER GP 100: Because of legal problems stemming from accidental
shootings, the double-action (DA) revolver remains popular in certain
circles, including many police departments, some of which have the
single-action (SA) capability removed by their department gunsmith.*

kill you. He now has the opportunity. You feel you're in jeopardy. So? Why not cast away all you've learned about self-defense and run? The court will surely ask, "Could you not have extricated yourself from all of this woe by simply making a hasty retreat?"

The problem is, some places in the world allow you to defend yourself in such a situation. Others are not so lenient. They require that you make an attempt to retreat.

How do they define retreat? Many locals say only if the retreat can be accomplished without putting you or innocents in danger.

Again, we turn to English common law, which states: "A man's home is his castle, and if attacked inside he is not required to retreat." (Remember this does not apply to the street, which is clearly not your castle.) Even the English common law on your home clearly states that there must be a clear and significant threat to yourself and those within your home before you can justifiably use deadly force. You cannot kill an intruder in your home for the mere fact he broke into said home. So, we are back where we started, aren't we? Even in your home, an attempt at retreat is a good idea, especially if you have a safe room from which you can telephone the police. More on the safe room in Chapter 8.

AFTER LETHAL FORCE IS USED

All right. That street punk left you no choice. Hopefully, he's now roasting on a spit in hell. You are now being investigated. What to do? What not to do? Jonathan, our former American street cop and SWAT team member, tells me the following things to look out for at this stage.

Never Tell a Lie

Lying will get you into trouble since if you go to trial the lie will be used as a weapon against you no matter how much you attempt to explain why you did it. You will be labeled a liar, and anything you say after that will be suspect.

Do Not Run Away

Running away will be seen as a confession of guilt. We all see an innocent man as one who is ready to stand trial to clear his good name. Doing the opposite casts a dark shadow on your defense. Don't panic, stand your ground; it's the best defense.

Do Not Tamper with the Evidence

The old ploy about a cop using a "throwaway" gun to make it seem the person he shot was armed is almost a sure ticket to prison in itself on a charge of obstruction of justice and goes a long way in casting a suspicion of murder on you. The same goes for dragging the body into your home and placing a kitchen knife in its hand. All this is a felony in itself. These kinds of ideas circulate in the street; avoid them at all cost.

Don't Have "Diarrhea of the Mouth"

All police officers know that questioning a suspect right after a crime is allegedly committed catches the suspect at his most weak moment. This is the time you may be in shock. This is the time you may be most susceptible to suggestion no matter how innocently it is rendered. You will want to justify what you did to all who are within range. You may be a witness against yourself and, considering the emotion of the moment, a very damaging witness at that. Shut your mouth. Call a lawyer; talk to him. If you must speak, say, "He attempted to murder me. I want my lawyer present before I go into more detail." Whatever you say, don't say, "I shot the S.O.B.," or something similar.

Lawyers Can Be Liars

My friend Hanon used to fracture the English language by calling lawyers "liars." He couldn't pronounce the word lawyer. He may have had a point. Remember, once in court, the prosecution will use all means legal and immoral to get you. If you insist in walking around in cammo and wearing a T-shirt with the words "Born to Kill" emblazoned across it, don't be surprised if it's considered "prior intent" by the prosecution. Use not-so-common sense—the life you save may be your own.

The American jurist Oliver Wendell Holmes wrote in a 1921 Supreme Court decision: "Detached reflection cannot be demanded in the presence of an uplifted knife." He was right, but these are the crazy 1990s, and anything goes.

STREET SURVIVAL LESSONS

1) *Know the law.* The time to learn the laws of self-defense in your jurisdiction is best before the fact and not after.

2) *Plan law scenarios.* Have scenarios worked out that apply to laws on the use of deadly force so that you don't over or underreact in a potential or actual violent encounter.

3) *You are innocent; act like it.* Create scenarios for how you would act after using deadly force. Remember, you are a law-abiding person who was forced to use justifiable force in defense of life. You are innocent of criminal intent. Act like it. The correct mind-set is just as important after you use deadly force as before.

Chapter Two

Know
Thine Enemy

*I*t's an old axiom that to emerge successfully from any contest, be it war, sport, or personal combat, you should know your enemy. You should be aware of his strong and weak points so that you can capitalize on them, persevere, and win. Ignorance can kill you when you are the target of an aggressor. On the other hand, knowledge can be a key component of victory when you are called upon to defend your life against attack. Who are the adversaries you may be called upon to duel out on the street? Are they just criminals, or are they as diverse as mankind itself? To give us a better perspective, it might be helpful to categorize them according to type.

THE PROFESSIONAL CRIMINAL

The professional criminal has been portrayed at his very best in numerous Hollywood films as the sophisticated and handsome cat burglar who has women fawning over him while he chooses a bottle of rare bubbly from a wine list. The quasi hero, always in control—crime is almost easy for him. He considers it a duel of wits between himself and the law. We have seen such a character excuse himself from the table, go upstairs to lift millions in jewelry out of a safe, careful not to hurt anyone but the insurance company, then return to the table in time to sample the wine, not a drop of sweat on his brow, not a single hair out of place. He is calm, cool, collected, almost a likable knave, since like Robin Hood he only robs the very rich and does it with such panache.

This may be a very unrealistic picture of the professional criminal, but it does have some elements of truth. These types of criminals are usually nonviolent. Most refuse to carry any sort of weapon, let alone a firearm. More than willing to face burglary charges, they are not stupid enough to let themselves be open to charges of aggravated assault, armed robbery, or murder.

Such criminals are usually not interested in petty crimes and so avoid lower- and middle-class homes like the plague. The prize available in such abodes is simply not worth the candle. These criminals are specialists who prey on the rich. Most of us will probably never have any contact with these types, for they operate in a quite rarefied social and economic strata.

There is an even more sophisticated type in this genre, one who specializes in the hardest of all crimes to detect: white collar crime. These are the "inside traders"—the stock scam operators, and so on. We can meet these types if we are in business or play the stock, bond, or commodity markets. They hover over these markets like flies over garbage, but they are hard to detect.

The one thing we must keep in mind about all of these so-called professional criminals is that they tend to be nonviolent. They hurt your wallet severely, but rarely your body—that is unless you are prone to heart attack or ulcers. Nevertheless, they do not go around with a sign around their necks proclaiming that they are nonviolent pros. Because of this and the fact that they, like any human being, are still prone to panic under stress, they must be treated with caution.

STREET SURVIVAL LESSON

1)   *A criminal is a criminal*. While certain elite groups of criminals tend to be less violent than others, it still behooves one to treat any suspect with maximum alertness and caution, since there are no guarantees he might not panic and use deadly force.

THE RANK AMATEUR

The amateur is potentially a very dangerous criminal in that his very inexperience makes him edgy and vulnerable to panic under pressure. He almost always is armed with a deadly though not very sophisticated weapon. A knife or a cheap handgun is his usual choice. The amateur rarely plans things out to the end like the professional does. Rather, he is usually an opportunist, taking advantage of a situation without prior thought or proper planning. The amateur makes decisions on the spur of the moment, sometimes under severe pressure and in a growing panic. Killing you or not is just another one of his hasty decisions.

Police officers usually find it easier to track this type of criminal down since he makes mistakes, sometimes very foolish ones. For example, a very publicized act of foolishness was in the World Trade Center bombing when one of the suspects went back to get his $400 deposit on a car used in the crime. He was the weak link in the conspiracy—a rank amateur whose stupidity resulted in the case being cracked and the apprehension of a slew of more professional terrorist criminals.

STREET SURVIVAL LESSON

1)   *Beware the amateur criminal*. The amateur can be

compared to an unguided missile that contains a deadly warhead. The path he chooses puts everyone around him in jeopardy.

....

THE PSYCHOPATH

The psychopath, unlike the amateur, usually has a plan. The problem is the plan usually makes sense only to him. In tracking down psychopaths, detectives try to detect a tell-tale pattern to their crimes. There usually is one, though it may be very difficult to trace. These may be the so-called serial killers, killers who are bent on eliminating some particular members of society. In Victorian England, "Jack the Ripper" made it his business to murder street prostitutes. In our time, "Son of Sam" heard voices and decided to murder innocent young women. Their psychosis spurred them on. To paraphrase Shakespeare, "There is a method to their madness."

Temporary Insanity: The Instant Psychopath
Another phenomenon of our time has been the seemingly normal person who suddenly flips and proceeds to shoot everyone down in a single episode of temporary madness. These instant psychopaths behave like a supersaturated solution—one drop more of whatever irritates them crystallizes and is enough to set them off.

These types have appeared on highways, where even a minor alleged insult triggers them off, resulting in death and mayhem.

Robotic Determination
The psychopath has a single-mindedness about him that makes him seem almost impervious to bullets. He resembles a robot who is programmed to do a certain task. These creatures, when on the rampage, are very difficult to stop since only a hit that shuts down their central nervous system will suffice. Against these types, a 12-gauge shotgun loaded with 00 buck may seem totally inadequate, for unless the central

nervous system or a major leg bone is hit, they don't go down. Peripheral hits, even with shotguns, may not do the trick.

....

STREET SURVIVAL LESSON

1) *Shoot straight.* Because of the increasing prevalence of psychopathic behavior by the criminal element of society, one should not only focus on obtaining a larger caliber, improved bullet design, or increased magazine capacity. What is needed is a serious return to good marksmanship. Bullet placement is more critical than it ever was. A good rule of thumb is to aim for the center of mass for distances beyond a half yard and at close-to-contact distance for head shots.

....

THE DRUG ADDICT

Many experts claim that hard-core drug addicts are not true criminals in the usual sense of the word but sick people who desperately need treatment for their malady. Unfortunately, the person assaulted by one of these "walking patients" in the street has a difficult time making such a humane diagnosis.

It's hard to believe that some of us can actually remember a more tranquil time in history when the use of hard drugs was simply not a factor in daily life. There was some reference to it in literature, but generally the public was unaware except to associate it with arty bohemian types who frequented some of the unsavory parts of town. Such is not the case today. Suffice to say there is hardly a community anywhere that does not have its drug addiction problems—problems which are growing daily. Drug addiction supports what is supposedly one of the biggest businesses in the world today. Some say the drug trade racks up more than $250 billion in street sales in the United States alone each and every year and is one of the few businesses that never experiences a recession, let alone a depression.

The time when we could avoid the fallout of drug addiction is past. Today, it is probably the greatest single cause of street crime in the world. Addicts with habits that cost them hundreds if not thousands of dollars a day must get money by any and all means possible. You and your family are their primary targets. They are dangerous, more dangerous than just about any criminal since there is a desperation in their crimes—a desperation borne of the fear of not having their "fix."

Addicts high on drugs have become the bane of law enforcement officers. Like the psychopath, nay, maybe even more since their presence on the streets is so common today, they have increased our desire for greater stopping power. This has created a boom market for handgun bullets that push back the state-of-the-art in bullet construction as we climb the expansion ladder, seeking more and more caliber and higher capacity in an attempt to give the officer of the law and the law-abiding citizen a chance when facing these junkies. Like with the psychopathic robot, a junkie high on drugs may become impervious to bullets. At last count, I read that 33 Winchester Power Points in 9mm Parabellum (9mmP) failed to stop one of these human sponges. I am quite sure the record is near to being or has already been surpassed at this writing.

STREET SURVIVAL LESSON

1) *First-shot placement is critical.* Like the psychopath, the drug addict must be taken down by good shot placement. The first bullet is extremely important since the body seems to increase its tolerance to subsequent hits as long as these hits are not into the brain or spine. Merely chopping-up flesh doesn't work.

There once was a time when street gangs were personified by such film staples as the Dead End Kids and the Bowery Boys. As the saying goes, "We've come a long way, baby." Street gangs today are sometimes better armed than the local police. They made the phrase "high capacity" a household word and have made the high-capacity craze grow by leaps and bounds as some of us feel the need for pistol, rifle, and shotgun filled to the brim with lethal projectiles. Whether all street gangs are so-armed is a moot question; the media have convinced the public they are.

The street gangs of today spend much of their time fighting one another for control of the local drug trade. The infamous "drive-by shooting" is an inevitable outcome of greed and the utter lack of morality. Time was when shooting a child in one of these drive-by killings was enough to get you hated by all, including the local underworld. Those days are long gone. Crime today may be organized at the higher levels, but out on the street it still is somewhat disorganized. Therefore, the chance of getting yourself or your family hurt in one of these street assassinations is growing daily. The number of well-armed gangs on the local scene is growing by leaps and bounds.

STREET SURVIVAL LESSON

1) *High-capacity is favored.* High-capacity can now be obtained without sacrificing caliber and shot placement. The days of two- to three-bullet gun fights are receding into history in some parts of the world.

DEVIL AND OTHER CULTS

Another sign of our times is the growth of cults, some of them with deadly philosophies that resemble the most infamous Indian Cult on the subcontinent, "the Thuggies." The

Thuggies used to strangle their hapless victims. The word thug is directly related to their onerous activities. In the film *Gunga Din*, Cary Grant came upon one such group of hundreds who were about to commit human sacrifice to the god Kali. When caught, Grant uttered one of those classic gems that make cinemagraphic history: "You're all under arrest!"

Unfortunately, the hapless victims who have fallen into the hands of these modern-day thugs usually have not had the luck to survive and tell the tale. Devil worship is a fast-growing cult which many times has animal and human sacrifice as part of its bizarre rituals. Torture of the most horrible nature usually precedes the immolation of the victim.

Some police officers quietly warn that many missing people—children included—have been the victims of such cults who hunt people in the streets like predators in the jungle. They are not above using methods other than force to snare their hapless victims. Some of their methods are quite ingenious, taking advantage of people in distress, lonely people, or the young and gullible. Some may act the role of the Good Samaritan, being most helpful in their attitude toward the needy and the unsuspecting. I remember a recent case where human and animal bones were found across the U.S. border in Mexico. Unsuspecting college students had disappeared. The devil-worshipping cult was led by a prim female school teacher, if memory serves me right. The usual "I can't believe she would do that; she was so nice" words were chanted by friends who saw her on TV.

Street survival against these types is based largely on cultivating and acquiring a very keen alley cat type of outlook on life. Suspicion of people, even "nice, friendly people," helps you and your family survive. Teaching children this unpleasant fact of life is critical. Devil cults especially like children for their rituals.

....

STREET SURVIVAL LESSON

1) *Be skeptical of do-gooders.* Be careful when

approached by people that are just too friendly and nice to be real. They may not be.

....

STATE-SPONSORED TERRORISM

With the demise of Soviet communism, many people breathed easier in the mistaken belief that state-sponsored terrorism would be on the decline around the globe. The opposite has proven true. Growing and highly dangerous types of state-sponsored terrorism have been spawned in the Mideast; Iran, Syria, Iraq, Sudan, and Libya have been the breeding grounds.

The best way to understand what may eventually be a very real and deadly problem in street survival is to actually read the words of the leaders of Islamic terrorism, understanding as we read them that these words are taken as the ultimate truth and blueprint for actions by hundreds of millions of true believers.

Sheik Omar Abdel-Rachman, a spiritual leader who was detained in New York in 1993 for his role in the World Trade Center bombing, wrote a turgid biography, *A Word of Truth* (which should be required reading for all law enforcement officers). His advice to so-called "lovers of truth": "Hit hard and kill the enemies of God in every spot to rid it of the descendants of apes and pigs. . . . There is no truce in the Islamic holy war against the enemies of Allah."

The good lover of truth offers some more gems for Moslem youth to follow: "Some people say the Christians are good people. . . . They are not. They are evil. They pretend because they want to spread their false beliefs. They are the enemy."

Unfortunately, old axioms die very slow deaths. The idea of domestic terrorism directed at the United States by a world network of Islamic fanatics still seems far-fetched for most Americans to accept even at this writing—even after the murder of Rabbi Meir Kahana in New York, even after the World Trade Center bombing. America, insulated and isolat-

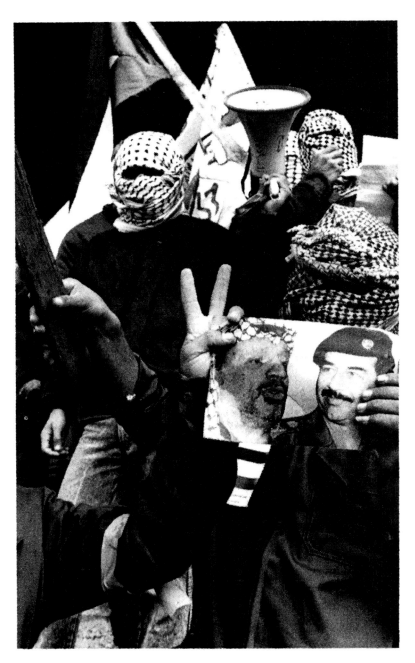

STATE-SPONSORED TERRORISM.

ed for so many years from such horrors, still looks over its borders, and not within them, for enemies. Progress and education are slow, but beginning.

The Superterrorist

Easily transported weapons of mass destruction have opened up a new world of possibilities for the individual terrorist bent on causing mass casualties. In the near future, we may face suitcase nuclear bombs, airborne attacks that spew forth deadly anthrax, chemical additions to our drinking water and food, and terrorist attacks on vital and potentially dangerous installations.

The United States Nuclear Regulatory Commission has recently decided that a new program for protecting vulnerable nuclear power plants from truck-bomb attacks will be implemented. We must remember that the hundreds of U.S. Marines killed and maimed in Beirut by such terrorists were murdered by such trucks laden with high explosives.

Plastic explosives developed in the former communist state of Czechoslovakia and given to Libya's Mohammed Gadaffi are usually the explosives of choice, though a homemade chemistry set type of fertilizer-based explosive was concocted for the World Trade Center bombing. This bodes ill for the future, because it means that individuals can do unprecedented damage to life and property from basic ingredients available on any farm or plant nursery.

The world of the superterrorist has dawned. Is the world ready for this? At this writing, I believe not. Can you, the individual bent on surviving in the street, do anything about it? I believe so.

Economic Targets

The militants seem to be selecting targets that are of an economic nature. The World Trade Center bombing cost close to $1 billion in damage and lost business. In Egypt, attacks on foreign tourists are occurring almost daily.

Tourism is an important source of hard currency for Egypt, critical to the economic survival of a nation that

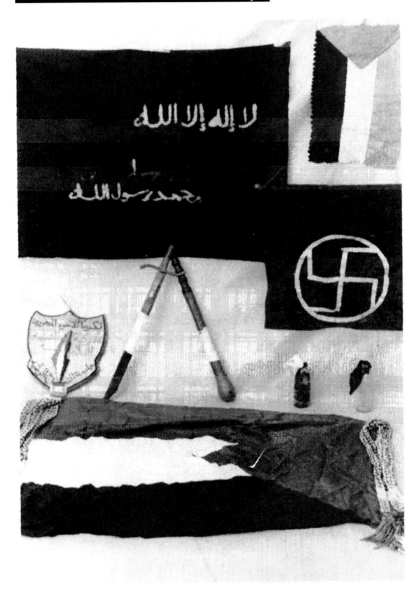

SYMBOLS OF TERROR FLOCK TOGETHER: *The Nazi swastika and the symbol of an Arab terror group sit side by side in this hideout.*

increases its population by more than a million people a year. The militants know this and so have gone for its jugular vein: the economy.

"Khomeini Moros"—The Islamic Fundamentalists

From Iran, a deadly new form of state-sponsored terror is pouring out over the globe, bringing in its wake murder and destruction. The Islamic fundamentalists' target is clear, their potential victims forewarned: you and I. They have declared a war to the death against the "Great Satan" (The United States of America) and "Little Satan" (Israel). Along with these targets can be added the secularist Arab states in the Middle East as well as Western Europe.

It is my personal belief that the phenomena of militant Islam renewed, something I first wrote about ("Hitler on the Gulf—A Scenario on the Consequences of the Iranian Revolution," *Counterpoint*, Jan. 1987, pp. 42-46, and a two-part article, "Fanaticism and the 1990s Battlefield," *Defense Update International*, Part 1: 1900–1950, No. 82, July-Aug. 1987, pp. 42-46 and Part 2: 1950–1990s, No. 85, pp. 6-8), poses a growing threat to personal survival in the streets.

The doctrine of religious hatred may grow like a cancer even in the unlikely environment of North America. Living in Israel, I was not surprised when I heard about the bombing of the World Trade Center. On the contrary, what amazed me and many observers over here was that such acts had not taken place before in North America. How could a doctrine of equating America with Satan not give rise to cruel violence and death of innocent Americans? Well, the evil genie is out of the bottle; militant Islam has picked up the sword of the Crusades. The average American—and the world as we know it—may never be the same. I shudder to think of what is in the cards if an unholy alliance is formed by them and the street gangs that infest some of the large urban centers of North America. The seed of international terrorism is attempting to sprout in main street U.S.A.

STREET SURVIVAL LESSON

1) *High-risk targets.* Islamic Fundamentalists can be expected to target economic and financial targets in North America. While there is little that individuals can do about this except to avoid them, law enforcement agencies should take precautionary measures. Even a small police department should be aware of what almost certainly will be a growing threat.

YOUR OWN INTERNAL ENEMY?

We have described external enemies and categorized them for easier understanding. We would be remiss not to add one other potential enemy to the list. Since this book is dedicated to helping you survive out there in the street, it would be wrong of me *not* to write of an internal potential enemy who could get you in a lot of needless trouble—you.

Concentrating on our handling of threats can sometimes blind us to a very important point. We must also know when it is prudent to hold back and not react to provocation. That is also a needed skill. Most people interested in what (for lack of a better term) we'll call self-defense are reactive types. These are people who do not shirk from provocation but are willing to do battle. For them to do otherwise is a gesture viewed as something akin to cowardice. Because of this mind-set, probably the hardest thing to teach such individuals is the need to back away and not do battle.

We must keep in mind the simple fact that not all provocations are in need of a verbal or physical response. That it is indeed true at times when the greatest sign of strength is the need to avoid confrontation. This is not to say that one must accept physical abuse, only that one must not initiate a counterattack when one is not actually in physical danger or under physical attack. Verbal abuse by an enemy does not always have to be answered in kind. Verbal abuse by an adversary does not have to escalate into a physical encounter. Old Teddy Roosevelt's saying, "Speak softly and carry a big stick," is probably the most difficult thing you may have to do, but probably the wisest. I interviewed Schlomo Baum on this seemingly somewhat different aspect of street survival:

E.S.: Do you have any examples in mind pertaining to the need to at least attempt to avoid conflict when out on the street?

S.B.: Many. However, two episodes come to mind that have many elements and which I believe may be of interest.

E.S.: Is one of them that incident with that Arab construction worker in Jerusalem? I forgot the details.

S.B.: Yes.

Case Study: Tire Slasher

S.B.: As you know, finding a parking space in Jerusalem, like in many other cities around the world, is becoming increasingly difficult. I spotted a space near a construction site and swung into it. I jumped out and was proceeding to lock the door when a construction worker ran up to me and told me that I couldn't park there.

E.S.: What did you say?

S.B.: I looked around in surprise and told him that there was not any signs, city or private, that said the space was closed to cars.

E.S. What did he say to that?

S.B.: He said he didn't need a sign. He decided it was closed.

E.S.: Was he armed in anyway?

S.B.: No. I told him that he could not close a public parking space at his whim. He had more than enough room around the construction site for trucks to use. At this, his eyes narrowed and he looked at me in a very unfriendly manner. I smiled and walked from the car. Then it happened.

E.S.: He pulled a weapon?

S.B.: He was too smart for that. No. He just asked me if

my car's tires were expensive and if I would like to find them slashed when I returned.

E.S.: What did you do then? Kick his ass?

S.B.: No. I walked to the car, got in, drove off, and looked for another parking space.

E.S.: That seems slightly out of character for you.

S.B.: On the contrary. Never fight a battle you have no chance of winning if you can avoid it. Never physically escalate a verbal exchange. What he said to me was not heard by others. If I had attacked him I would have been in the wrong as far as the law is concerned. The parking area was near the construction site. He could have claimed in court that he needed it. The whole basis of the dispute was therefore not crystal clear. Better to leave and find another parking space. I have enough self-confidence to do that. He was smirking, but I decided not to wipe it off of his face. Now, let's speak about another example of attempting to avoid conflict.

Case Study: Baum on the Bus

S.B.: A few years ago, I had gone to Haifa, as you know, a northern port city here in Israel. I was patiently waiting at the head of a long line of tired-looking bus passengers for the bus to Jerusalem to arrive, when a noisy gang of five street punks in their early twenties walked up. They were seeing off their leader, a tough-looking fellow. He stepped to the front of the line, right in front of me as if I and the others didn't exist.

E.S.: What did you do?

S.B.: I gently tapped him on the shoulder and pointed out that the line formed at the rear. He stared at me with disbelief and utter contempt. Obviously, the soft-spoken elderly gentleman, pipe in mouth and newspaper in hand, wasn't worth bothering with, and he continued laughing with his friends. I again gently tapped his shoulder and informed him, pointing to the rear of an increasingly longer line, where the line formed. He in no uncertain terms informed me where I could go and turned back to his friends. I again gently tapped his shoulder and this time informed him not to try to board the bus ahead of us all when it pulled up since he was in the wrong. He once again informed me of the fact that he held me in the lowest disregard. By this time the other bus passengers were quite convinced I was about to obtain the beating of my life and motioned for me to back off.

E.S.: What happened next?

S.B.: The bus pulled up. Its door swung open, and the young punk escalated the encounter. He crossed the invisible red line. He smashed his elbow into me and started to come up with a punch. I deftly side-stepped, keys in hand, key points sticking out like a Roman celestis, and plunged them into his cheek, slicing him open like a can of tuna. Blood spurted all over the bus as he fell back into his buddies' arms.

E.S.: What did you do?

S.B.: I climbed into the bus, calmly walked to the back, sat down, placed my unlit pipe in my mouth and nonchalantly proceeded to read the newspaper. Suddenly, I was disturbed by a loud clamor. It seems that a mini-riot had broke out. The bus driver, the bleeding punk, his gang, and the shocked passengers milled around in utter confusion, shouting loudly. I looked up to see a somewhat berserk man charge onto the bus and make for me. He screamed, "What's going on! I am a member of Knesset [Israel's Parliament]! I am a member of Knesset!"

E.S.: What did you say to that? I mean, he has legal immunity, sort of like an unofficial prosecutor or something.

S.B.: "Sir, I don't blame you one bit. Why, if I was a member of Knesset, I would shout it aloud in the streets and buses, too. It's a wonderfully well paying job, so many perks and benefits."

E.S.: What happened next?

S.B.: Two police officers ran onto the bus, quite agitated since they thought that a member of Parliament had been attacked. When he informed them that the street punk holding his bloody T-shirt to his face was the victim, their ardor melted. I proceeded to inform them of the true facts.

E.S.: That you hit the punk?

S.B.: No. That I was attacked by a gang of ruffians whose leader came at me when I tried to board the bus. Blind luck was with me and he slipped. It was obvious that he must have cut his face on the side of the door. Why, if it weren't for that I probably would have been beaten to a pulp or worse. "I'm on the elderly side," I gingerly informed them, very afraid that I would be brutally attacked after the police left. I demanded police protection.

E.S.: Did you get police protection?

S.B.: Most certainly. The police officers walked over to the bleeding punk and his gang and asked for IDs. [The officers] then told them that if any of them tried to take revenge on me they would be in big trouble. At this the gang left and the bleeding young punk sat down a few seats in front of me. As the bus proceeded down the coastal highway, I rose and walked over to him. I gently tapped him on the shoulder. This time he looked at me quite differently from how he did on the bus platform. I smiled and softly asked him a question, but he didn't give me a reply.

E.S.: What was the question?

S.B.: I asked him, "Do you like what I did? Would you like to turn the other cheek so that I can do the other side?"

....

STREET SURVIVAL LESSONS

1) *Never physically escalate a verbal encounter.* Words alone are not cause enough for a physical response, especially when those words allude to something that may happen in the future.

2) *"A stitch in time saves nine."* When the situation allows and you have decided not to back off, give your adversary a clear, nonbelligerent warning that his actions are not going to be tolerated. Though Baum did place his finger on the young punk's shoulder, it was done in such a gentle manner that it did not elicit a violent response.

3) *Give your enemy a chance to retreat.* Baum did

leave open an avenue of escape for the young punk to move through. However, Baum was faced with a matter of principle, a clear need to stop this gang from intimidating the people in line.

4)   *Nonweapons can be weapons.* Using his keys as a weapon, he became armed in a manner that shifted the odds in his favor should the gang attack, but not be seen as being armed if he had to undergo a body search. (We review the use of keys as a street weapon in Chapter 3.)

5)   *Anticipate your enemies' tactics.* He expected the attacker to lunge at him, so he side-stepped and countered with the keys, which he then slipped into his pocket without anyone, including the punk leader and his gang, seeing. They were dumbfounded as to what exactly had occurred.

6)   *Stay cool.* By going to the rear of the bus and sitting down to read his paper, Baum added to the confusion of all concerned as to exactly what had really happened. He didn't shout or run away. He was not guilty of breaking the law, and he acted that way.

7)   *Grasp psychological opportunities.* Seeing that the police officers were less concerned with the street gang than they were with the idea of a member of Parliament being attacked, Baum immediately went on the psychological offensive, cleverly playing the role of the frightened elderly gentleman. It worked. Case closed.

....

NOTE: The psychological ploy of rubbing what happened into the bleeding street punk when he was alone on the bus is not recommended as a street survival tactic, nor is stretching the truth about what really happened when relating the story to the police (unless, of course, you are cut from the same fabric as Baum).

Case Study: Tent of Hospitality

Timing is everything in financial investment. It is also important when one is faced with danger. The ability to use correct timing is critical to one's physical survival. Simply attacking when you are in danger may not be the prudent thing to do at all times. Sometimes, knowing one's enemy, his customs, etc., allows you to wait for the opportune moment to strike. The following case study is such a case.

Eddie (our former Korean War vet) tells of an incident that occurred when he tangled horses in the hills and valleys on the fringes of Israel's southern desert, the Negev.

Now we must keep in mind that Eddie comes from good stock. His great uncle Sam Driben has a statue of himself near El Paso. Seems he served as a scout for Black Jack Pershing when he raided into Mexico going after Poncho Villa. Sam was an expert dynamiter who had learned his trade in Mexico during their revolution and knew the back country well.

Eddie's father, Irv Driben, joined the U.S. Marines when he was 16, serving in just about every U.S. war in the so-called banana republics, as well as the Boxer Rebellion, and who later was police chief of both St. Petersburg and Clearwater, Florida. He originally aspired to joining the French Foreign Legion, hoping to fight the Riffs of North Africa, but ruined that opportunity after he smelled the perfume on the French recruiting officer and proceeded to punch him out for being a sissy. After that he demanded to know where the hell the Riff recruiting office was. He wasn't going to serve under any pansy who used perfume. Irv was disappointed to be informed there wasn't any Riff office.

E.S.: Eddie, you mentioned to me you had a good yarn about how knowing thine enemy helped save your life.

E: It was a particularly tense time. Egyptian commandos

were in the Negev desert, and fighting was going on all around the area. Wrangling horses had put me in contact with the Bedouin tribes who moved across the borders of Israel, Jordan, and the Egyptian Canal. I had got to know a member of one small tribe quite well.

E.S.: Could you describe him for us?

E: His name was Ahda. He spoke good English. He was special. His rifle was in first-class condition, as was the knife he always carried. He wasn't like the others.

E.S.: You mean they didn't take care of their equipment? I thought in the movies the wild nomadic tribes lived with their weapons in hand?

E: They do, but that don't mean they take good care of them. Anyway, I was scouting the hills for pasture and decided to pay a visit to the tent of the tribe's sheik who was Ahda's brother. When I pulled back the flap and entered, I saw Ahda's brother, who gave me a scared look. He looked nervous as hell.

E.S.: Was Ahda there?

E: No. But, sitting in the tent were three men who did not look Bedouin. Their skin was lighter, and they were slender, just looked different. In a split second I realized they were Egyptians—well-armed Egyptians with FN pistols and rifles. They were smugglers who evidently used the tribes.

E.S.: What were you armed with?

E: I had a rifle and a knife. Left my damn pistol at home. I instantly knew I'd regret that—if I lived.

E.S.: I don't understand. You had a rifle?

E: The custom is that once I entered the tent I was under the protection of the sheik's hospitality. I, like the Egyptians, was obliged to sit on the rugs, slowly sip coffee, and eat. All rifles were placed behind us. That meant they had pistols and I only had a small Bowie knife that I had made for myself. Three of them armed with pistols and me with a knife. Miserable odds.

E.S.: Maybe they weren't hostile.

E: No such luck. After the sheik told me to sit, which I did as far away from them as I could, they proceeded to kill me with their eyes, giving me looks of deep hatred. They snickered between themselves in Arabic (I understood the language) about the Jews. I realized I had probably made a fatal mistake.

E.S.: By going into the tent.

E: Of course. How was I going to get out of this alive? In the tent, seated and sipping Turkish coffee, the chances were they wouldn't break the hospitality code of the desert and kill me. But once I got up to leave and reached for my rifle, that code might not stick with them. After all, they were city Egyptians, not Bedouin. That was easy to see. I could smell life or death hanging in the air.

E.S.: You must have been scared.

E: Some, but I'm not just afraid of dying. What I am afraid of is dying and not taking enough of my enemies with me. Hell, if I have to die, why not them, too? If I die, so do they. It was then that I realized I had made a worse mistake. So I made up my mind to fix that.

E.S.: What mistake?

E: Hell, they had pistols and I had a knife. Why sit far from them? One knife is only good at close quarters. I figured if I could get close to them I could at least kill two of them before the third one shot me.

E.S.: But isn't that against the code of the desert? The tent, coffee, and all? Desert hospitality?

E: When it comes to survival I have my own code. Screw the code of the desert.

E.S.: What could you do? You already were seated.

E: Well, for the next two hours I moved, inch by inch, toward them. All the time we sipped and sipped and stared at each other while the sheik looked like he was going to faint. Just about one second before I was going to pull my knife, Ahda pulled back the tent flap and came in. He gave me a look and then proceeded to shake everyone's hand. Then he reached down and pulled me slowly out of the tent while he smilingly made small talk.

E.S.: What happened then?

E: I got on my horse and he got on his camel and we made

quick tracks for the desert. He said that the second he walked into that tent he sensed what was happening. Says he knew I was gonna slice his brother's visitors up like shish kebab, and figured he'd better get me out of there. I told him I had never been so happy to see someone in my life. We had a good laugh and went out scouting for new pasture.

....

STREET SURVIVAL LESSONS

1) *Timing is everything.* Sometimes it may pay to wait, even though you may want to react. Eddie has a good sense of timing. He didn't attack but rather tried to increase his survival odds by moving closer and closer to his enemies. In the end, he survived without having to attack.

2) *Know your enemy.* Know the customs of the potential enemies that frequent your area. Such knowledge just might save your life.

....

WORKING ALONE WITH POTENTIAL ENEMIES

One of the practical everyday problems many face around the world, and certainly in Israel, is the need to work alongside people who are potential enemies. Here the problem is very acute in the agriculture and the building trades. Most people don't realize that Israelis and Arabs interact in a positive manner on a day by day basis. The problem is that terrorists take advantage of this, waiting for the right moment to carry out a murderous attack. Personal security becomes very difficult. The problem of working with potential enemies seems to be increasing around the world as many nations find that the fragile tapestry holding religious and ethnic groups together begins to slowly unwind. The retribalization of the world is on the increase. Ethnic, racial, and religious strife is raising its ugly head.

I have been approached on numerous occasions by people facing quite difficult personal self-defense problems—problems which are compounded by the fact that they must work alone with their workers. An example would be farmers who work a small spread of land and are dependent on Arab workers to bring in crops that do not lend themselves to mechanization. This necessitates the farmers being alone in the field or in agricultural sheds with employees who are suspect as to their intentions.

Studying the problem, I have come up with what I believe are solutions that work, albeit difficult ones as far as the social interaction of worker and boss are concerned.

When using workers who are potential criminal terrorists, it *is* best to be very skeptical of any good past behavior record that the authorities give you vouching for a worker's lack of criminal intent. Many such people are clever moles who have infiltrated a work force. Others may be truly nonviolent types who have subsequently become unwilling but deadly killers, pressured by criminal terrorists to work for them. A recent terrorist attack was carried out by a long-trusted worker who said that the terrorists killed his youngest son and would continue to kill his children unless he did their bidding. His case was by no means a rare one. Having such a trusted worker on your payroll could prove even more dangerous because your guard would be down. That is why, for example, security services are constantly on the lookout for trusted workers in sensitive governmental positions who could be blackmailed or bribed into working for an enemy. Remember, if using potential enemies for laborers, such tricks of the trade could be used against you when you least expected it. Your worker could be targeted, not for spying, but for murder.

Better Safe than Sorry

When working with potential troublemakers, it is best to set the ground rules for the work procedure in a precise and clear manner at the very onset of the worker-boss relationship. Do not make up the rules as you go along. This signals that you are either afraid, confused, or both. Always tell such workers the ground rules, and do not back down in the face of protestations of innocence or nonviolent intentions. Do this in a firm, nonbelligerent manner, in a voice that does not telegraph anything else but a firm commitment to the rules.

If you are questioned as to the possibility of your rules being some sort of threat, I find honesty is the best policy. I say they are if they are broken. Being blunt can act as a deterrent. Facts, stated in a matter-of-fact manner, without any wavering, apologizing, or aggressiveness, are understood as simply stating the rules of the game.

I have advised lonely farmers who use contract workers to tell the workers never to come within 10 yards of them and to make it clear that breaking this iron rule will be considered a potentially hostile act. The 10-yard rule gives one the chance to respond to attack in that the distance is just outside the minimum 8-yard distance considered dangerous when facing a knife wielder. Remember, most workers, whether they be in construction or agriculture, are in excellent physical condition and have tools in their hands that have served as deadly close-quarter weapons for centuries. They can kill very efficiently. I can attest to this sad fact since hardly a week goes by here in Israel that this simple truth is not proven once again.

A GOOD DOG AND GUN

A good dog at your side is another street survival weapon that works on the job. If you can invest in a trained dog, all the better. The dog is probably worth as much as your gun, though I sincerely recommend having a gun, preferably a handgun, on your side that is always at hand and not leaning against a workbench. Don't be shy about displaying your handgun in its holster for all to ponder. Deterrence saves lives if it is credible. If you work a tractor or any loud equipment in the field, be forewarned that you are a very easy target for attack. Watching the ground and the work before you places you in a very difficult position. Also, the noise of the engine and other equipment serves to block out any sound of an approaching attacker. Many murderers around our parts have taken advantage of these facts. For drivers and operators of such equipment in the field or work shed, having a dog who is trained to be suspicious of anyone approaching you is a good idea. He'll do his job while you do yours, though do not rely on him alone. Placing mirrors around you, on your tractor, etc., helps you to be aware of anyone sneaking up.

Case Study: The Praying Tractor Driver

Yishi is a small agricultural settlement that lies in central Israel. It is populated by Israelis who originally came from Yemen or Morocco. A recent case of a Yemenite who drives a tractor and uses contract workers teaches us the value of always having a handgun on your person.

It seems that at the close of a workday in the fields, an altercation broke out between our tractor driver and some of his workers. The tractor driver told them that he would pay them for the day, but they didn't have to bother to show up for work the next morning. Then, as if by command, the six Arabs pulled long, razor-sharp butcher knives from under their loose-fitting shirts. One of them, a big burley fellow, grabbed the driver by the throat and hissed that he should prepare to meet his maker.

Knowing their culture very well, the driver asked that he be allowed to take a Bible he had stowed in a box on the tractor so that he could say a last prayer. All of them, being religious people, realized that the request was certainly not out of order. Our elderly tractor driver was allowed to get his Holy Bible. As he reached in for it, he grasped a small .380 auto. Turning to the knife wielders, he told them to throw down their weapons and raise their hands or they would meet their maker. This they did, since the grimly determined look on the weather-beaten face of the Yemenite tractor driver told them he was not a man given to idle threats. He then proceeded to march them to his house, where he called the police, who came and arrested the would-be killers.

After that little incident, our farmer tractor driver decided to carry his pistol on him. He still carries that Bible in that box on the tractor, claiming it saved his life just as certainly as that little .380.

Studying such incidents makes one see the value of not trusting potential troublemakers. Be it a cop on the beat or a prison guard in charge of convicted criminals, one has to be on full alert at all times and not fall prey to the very enticing theory that if one treats a man right, he'll do right by you, too. If you want to be loved, get a cocker spaniel. When working with potential enemies, criminals, or terrorists, it's better to be respected, nay, even feared, than succumb to what can only be called the deadly naiveté.

STREET SURVIVAL LESSONS

1) *A good dog.* Having a good dog when you work alone or with potential enemies is good survival insurance. While you work, they help you watch.

2) *Mirrors.* Have mirrors on your tractors, etc. that allow you to see anyone approaching you from the side or behind.

3) *A weapon on you.* Having a weapon that isn't on you could get you killed. Our tractor driver was lucky he was able to get to that box where his handgun was hidden. I have spoken to many farmers who did the same thing, hide a weapon in their car or tractor, worried that showing it would give off negative vibes to their workers. Have the weapon on you. To hell with the negative vibes.

4) *Lay out the ground rules.* When working with people you consider potentially dangerous, it is best to lay out the ground rules of your relationship at the outset in a clear manner.

5)   *10-yard rules.* Never let a potential enemy get closer to you than 10 yards when you are working with them. Consider this the absolute minimum distance. The further the better.

Chapter Three

Street Weapons— "Cold"

A rmed with a better understanding of what makes for a correct mind-set and infused with the knowledge of what type of enemies may await us out there on the street, we now must face the age-old problem of what weapons in our arsenal can be brought to bear and how these weapons should be handled so as to better ensure our survival in the street. In this chapter, we will deal with what the Israelis call "cold weapons," that is, weapons that are not firearms, or "hot weapons."

WHEN FIREARMS ARE FORBIDDEN

When writing such a book for world publication, one has to take into consideration the fact that in some places on this earth, legitimate self-defense weapons such as firearms in the hands of the law-abiding public are frowned upon by the very politicians who go around armed themselves and escorted by armed bodyguards to boot. I guess it depends on "whose bull is being gored."

They all seem to have one thing in common: utter contempt for their own people.

Can people denied firearms have alternative means of defeating street thugs? The answer lies in the use of cold weapons. A prerequisite for proper use of any weapon, and especially cold weapons, is a good general working knowledge of your primary target, the human body. The effective use of all weapons is substantially increased when you know which areas of the human anatomy are most susceptible to the weapon in hand, even if said weapon is, in fact, your hand. Trauma to the anatomical vital centers of the human body is the key to stopping power and lethality. And remember, with cold weapons a blow should be delivered with a blood-curdling battle cry so as to distract your enemy or throw him off stride.

VITAL ANATOMICAL TARGETS

The nervous system of the human body can be compared to a vast electrical power system—short it out and everything shuts down, sometimes for good. Experts agree unequivocally—a vital nerve area is the best target.

Vital Target #1: The Human Brain and Spine

The most vital areas of the nervous system are the human brain and spine. A hit that disrupts this vital area (sometimes called the T-Zone) is the fastest and surest way of incapacitating your adversary. The T-Zone, if penetrated or crushed by almost any bullet, bladed weapon, or blunt instrument, will shut down and short-circuit the vital central nervous system (CNS). Knowing the location of this vital target is critical to street survival. This "electrical system" is the number-one target; shutting it down is the number-one priority.

Vital Target #2: The Major Blood Vessels

Next in importance in target selection are the major blood vessels deep within the body. These are the vital conduits of life-sustaining blood. Piercing these "high-pressure hoses" can result in instant, massive hemorrhaging, rapid loss of blood pressure, and oxygen depletion of the brain, causing a massive shutdown of the central nervous system through the back door, so to speak, with fatal results. Bullets or blades do this.

Vital Target #3: The Lesser Blood Vessels

Slashing or piercing of the lesser blood vessels can result in a slower but no less dangerous shutdown of the body as the blood drains away. This phenomenon is known by all students of bladed weapons and is one of the principles of classical knife fighting.

Vital Target #4: Major Bones and Joints

Disruption of a major leg bone or leg joint can be critical to stopping your adversary from closing in on you. However, if your attacker is armed with a firearm or, for that matter, a crossbow, his attack could still be continued from afar. The human shoulder, elbow, knee, and hip joints are very susceptible. A blow or projectile delivered to any of these joints will put them out of action. Bullets, blades, or blunt weapon trauma will do the job.

Vital Target #5: The Eyes

The eyes are a very vulnerable target area—one, like the groin, that your enemy will protect instinctively. The most effective cold weapons against the eyes are aerosol spray weapons, especially those based on the use of red pepper. These have an effect lasting many minutes. Surprise weapons of opportunity, such as a handful of sand, coins, pebbles, etc., will also work, though they are less effective.

....

STREET SURVIVAL LESSONS

1)   *Battle cry.* All cold weapons should be delivered on target with a blood-curdling battle cry so as to distract one's enemy or throw him off stride.

2)   *Know your target.* A good working knowledge of

the human body and its vital centers is critical to the effective use of all weapons, and especially cold weapons. Picturing these vital centers in your mind should be automatic.

WEAPONS OF DISTRACTION

This category of "near weapons" ranges from a handful of coins to a chair thrown at an enemy. They are, of course, responses of opportunity, used when you have no other answer at hand and are in desperate need of distracting and slowing down an enemy's close-quarter attack. They have two goals: either to gain time so that you can draw a lethal weapon or, failing that, to retreat.

Handbag and Objects Within

I've watched numerous tapes on self-defense for women, and I usually turn them off, mumbling something like, "Now I've seen everything." Women are advised to carry oven cleaner in their handbags to ward off attack. Hair combs are deemed weapons. Hand mirrors are miraculously turned into deadly rapiers, ball-point pens into stilettos—the list is endless. The power to self-delude is never-ending. All of this nonsense can and does sometimes do one thing: it can get you quite killed.

How such items would work against a weight-lifting 260-pounder or an attack by the Savage Skulls cycle gang is anyone's guess. But in certain circles they are recommended as serious weapons rather than effective distracters or temporary incapacitators. Not surprisingly, courses that push these items as serious weapons usually open with an antigun lecture.

Now, let it be understood that I carry an aerosol can of pepper spray in my pocket when I travel, but I do not consider it a viable alternative to serious weaponry. It is there to handle or discourage a nonlethal confrontation. It is effective against irate people who are bent on conflict but do not warrant the use of more effective weapons. To seriously indoctrinate the unsuspecting and the naive into believing that they are the weapons of choice for warding off deadly attack is dangerous and borders on the criminal. They ought to ban these dangerous courses, not firearms.

Pocket Keys

In the chapter on the correct mind-set, I included a case study in which Schlomo Baum used an ordinary set of car keys as a weapon. This would seem to contradict what I have said about purse items used as weapons. It does not. In his mid-60s, Baum has a fist and a strength that far surpasses that of most men I know. The keys in his fist were in a stable vise that turned the whole unit into quite a formidable weapon. It was this formidable combination that elevated the keys into the realm of weaponry. If you have a strong hand, you will probably obtain the same results. If not, reader beware; the results may only serve to enrage your adversary even further.

....

STREET SURVIVAL LESSONS

1) *Know the true capabilities of each weapon.* Weapons of distraction or incapacitation should never be confused with serious weapons of self-defense.

2) *Don't believe in weapon fairy tales.* The misuse of nonweapons can get you maimed or killed.

....

The Martial Arts

The popularity of the martial arts was enhanced by such personalities as Bruce Lee in his now-classic films. Rooted in history, unarmed combat has been popular in Asia because the peasants were denied weapons. Answers were needed, and the growth of martial combat reached its zenith under such bizarre circumstances.

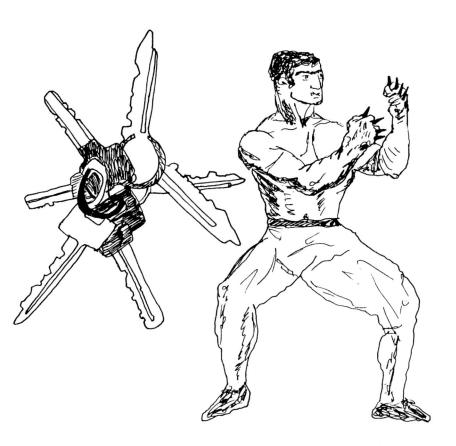

POCKET KEYS BETWEEN THE FINGERS: Pocket keys can be turned into formidable close-quarter weapons of surprise if you have powerful enough fists.

A student of these entertaining films will immediately see that our hero is almost never attacked by anyone carrying a firearm. If he is attacked by such an enemy, the enemy allows him to disarm him with almost monotonous regularity. Once our hero takes the firearm, he almost certainly tosses it aside with contemptuous disdain, refusing to soil his hands with such an unheroic weapon. As I mentioned, I very much enjoy such films, but I keep them in a compartment in my brain labeled "fantasy."

Now don't get your hackles up. I am not degrading the martial arts nor their practitioners. And I would most certainly not like to engage in martial combat with any of their masters. The fact is, I wouldn't like to engage any serious student of these arts, though I have engaged one or two not-so-serious ones and found them to be masters of the subject only in their heads and not in their hands.

Without a doubt, the martial arts of the Orient have captured the hearts and minds of much of the world. This is especially true when we realize how impractical boxing skills are for street survival. Karate, kung-fu, and the other oriental martial arts are certainly superior. Karate, which is taught in almost 5,000 schools across the United States alone, is presently the most popular. Reaching the eighth level of proficiency, the coveted black belt, is no mean achievement. Devotees who can smash boards or building blocks with *kara* (empty) *te* (hand) are not people you want to mess with. If you are someone who is disciplined enough to spend many months conditioning your body and up to three years to learn the ropes, you are exceptional; certainly you are not average.

Martial arts training can be very useful when your attacker is not considered to be of the life-threatening type. However, depending on the laws of the jurisdiction where you live, someone who uses martial arts skills against, say, a drunk at a bar, could be sued. The thin line between what is considered reasonable and excessive force works here, too.

Where martial arts training does do extremely well is in teaching one how to fend off a close-quarter attack within contact distance to one and one-half yards. Such skills may allow you to draw your handgun where others without your skills would fail.

The Combo Fighter

A martial arts expert who is a trained gunfighter is the most deadly combo we could face out there in the street. But the focus is on the word combo. I tend to be weapon oriented, and so are almost all of the serious practitioners of martial arts. In life-threatening situations, the combo approach is the ideal way to go.

Using your skills at close-quarter combat to disarm your armed opponent or throw him off balance so as to give you time to draw your weapon makes lots of street sense. The very best martial arts instructors believe in the combo approach.

STREET SURVIVAL LESSONS

1) *Martial arts skill alone may not work.* Understand that relying on the martial arts alone for street survival in this day and age can be detrimental to your health. Films are fantasy; the street isn't.

2) *The combo fighter is king.* Learn the martial arts with an eye toward coupling these skills with your firearms skills. The combo approach is the most deadly and life-saving partnership you can forge for street survival.

3) *Know your limitations.* Martial arts skill alone can be used very effectively against attackers not armed with deadly firearms. However, be careful not to be accused of the use of excessive force if you are a graduate of a martial arts school.

DIRTY FIGHTING

Whatever I have written for the use of the martial arts to protect human life goes for what is known as dirty fighting. However, for individuals who do not have the skill or patience to master any of the martial arts, there is, happily, this alternative.

A basic and crude form of the martial arts is dirty fighting. In dirty fighting, you really only learn a few basic moves and then rely on them if you do not have a weapon in hand or do not want to draw one. This form of hand-to-hand combat is dirty and unsportsmanlike. In dirty fighting, when your opponent is down, you see it as an opportunity to kick his brains out. There is nothing sportsmanlike about it, and it takes much, much less serious practice than, say, mastering karate. Again, it bears noting that karate and the other martial art forms are more effective than dirty fighting, but they take disciplined practice to acquire skills not easily pursued by the average and sometimes lazy individual. Dirty fighting techniques are for the less disciplined individual who just wants a few deadly pointers on how to finish an enemy fast and simple. It is also for the person who does not have a high degree of physical prowess and needs a practical, everyday, workable answer to street encounters that are not necessarily those in the realm of mortal combat.

The overriding principle of dirty street fighting is that anything goes. The object is to win. The dirty street fighter knows that one-punch knockouts rarely happen except on TV. He also knows that men who rely on their boxing skills can get crippled or killed by an enemy who is a master of dirty fighting.

The street fighter knows that his adversary's head is much harder than his fist and doesn't bother much with boxing. However, if you think you have the means of ending a fight with your fists or with those jujitsu moves you learned last week, try the following test, and remember that to engage in a real street fight you should be able to do the following on command:

    a) jog 1.5 miles and still be able to slowly drink a glass of water without shaking
    b) do a minimum of 30 deep knee bends and walk a straight line without swaying
    c) do a minimum of 30 push-ups without turning red-faced
    d) do a minimum 30 toe-touching bends without cheating

If you can do all of that, you probably will last about 90 seconds in a real street fight before you start weakening. If you cannot do all of the listed exercises, think twice before you engage in a real, prolonged street encounter.

Since many of us cannot pass these simple tests of stamina, we have to take into consideration the horrible fact that we probably won't last past 30 seconds in such an encounter and then will rapidly decline and deteriorate with resulting dangers. For the test failures, the best answers to winning a hand-to-hand combat situation in the street are the following.

Dirty Fighting Techniques

The cardinal rule: strike to vital targets (these are not the targets listed for knife fighting, etc.) that can be engaged by the human hand so as to damage and shut down vital body functions. A word of caution. Dirty fighting, like classical knife fighting in the "circle of death," is not for the squeamish.

Not everyone is willing to engage in it. Most people do not like the idea of actually feeling their enemy's anguish. That's why they prefer guns—they are so impersonal.

I remember seeing a young terrorist of about 17 on Israeli TV describe the joy he felt when his knife or ax plunged into his victims' bodies. He was an assassin for a PLO group that specialized in murdering Arabs who worked for and with Israelis. He liked slicing and chopping up his victims. He also relished performing these acts when his victims were tied down and after he had tortured them for days with bare electrical wires, gouged out their eyes, cut off their tongues, and castrated them. As I watched his smiling, innocent baby face, I realized what a severe disadvantage the normal, average person has in deadly combat with such creatures. He has a lot in common with psycho-murderers, spaced-out drug addicts, and sadistic killers. Try to remember that when you make a decision on how to defend yourself from these dregs of humanity. Unfortunately, they are not a rarity.

Being sportsmanlike and humane to such murderers can get you and your family butchered in a most brutal and cruel manner. They are out there in the street preying on the weak and unsuspecting.

Hanon once told me he had a firm principle of never falling

into the hands of the enemy. He and others had seen what some of them did to prisoners of war or kidnapped Israelis. With that chilling thought in mind, a few dirty fighting moves in our survival inventory may prove prudent afterall.

The Throat and Neck

The throat is a vital target and easily engaged by the human hand. Serious damage can result. This is a target for the man who relies on raw instinct and cunning rather than a repertoire of sophisticated blows learned and mastered only after a long and tedious program of practice and physical fitness.

The Adam's Apple

If any target could be called the ultimate one in dirty street fighting, it's the Adam's apple. It's a prominent target made by the cartilage of the larynx and is one that is not well-guarded by your enemy. Your opponent will not expect such an area to be attacked, and his guard may be down. If the Adam's apple is damaged, it can result in loss of speech and the ability to breathe. The pain felt is almost unbearable and is accompanied by choking and gagging. Any enemy so engaged will be deemed unfit to murder you, in short notice. It's a great fight stopper and guarantees you won't have to be pushed to the limit of your physical abilities. Incidentally, we once more remind ourselves that all blows delivered in this chapter are best accompanied by a very loud, blood-curdling battle cry.

Crippling Straight Blow

A blow to the Adam's apple is delivered by closing your hand back to the second finger joint. If you're right-handed, move forward with your left foot and smash upward with every bit of force you can muster with your right arm and shoulder. Aim for an area slightly above what is the base of the throat. If your aim is too low, it will be corrected by the sliding movement of your knuckles slamming up into your opponent's larynx.

Crippling Side Blow

If you cannot deliver a direct blow with the closed fist and knuckles, use a karate chop with the outside of your hand. This is best done by slightly crouching and then springing upward so that additional force is added to the blow, which is delivered by sweeping your arm up and backward in a powerful short arc.

Now here is where the dirty fighting reaches the moment of truth. Your opponent is down. Do you stand there and watch him groan? Do you help him up? Do you walk away? No, you certainly do not. Not in a dirty street fight.

Follow-Up Blows

You slam your shoe into his stomach, kick his head. Do it more than once. That should stop him from having any further notions of inflicting grave bodily harm on you. The follow-up blow is the critical factor in such encounters.

The Nose

Like all fighting, surprise is the key to success. Because the nose is nearer to the eyes than the larynx, it is instinctively better guarded. Still, it is not a target that people believe will be attacked directly in a rough-and-tumble street fight. What many do not know is that if the nose is struck with proper and well-directed force, it can end a fight there and then.

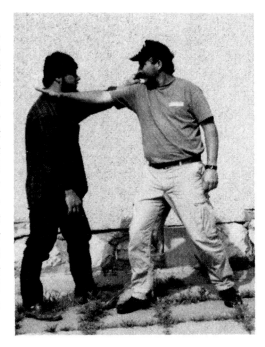

The Crippling Blow

Step forward with your left leg as

SIDE BLOW TO ADAM'S APPLE: Jonathan delivers a crippling side blow to his opponent's neck and Adam's apple.

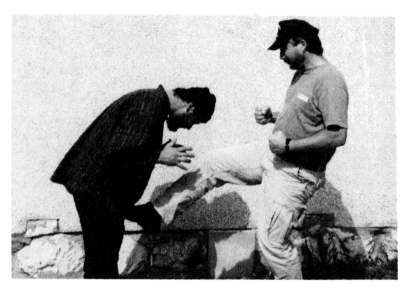

FOLLOW-UP KICK TO THE GROIN.

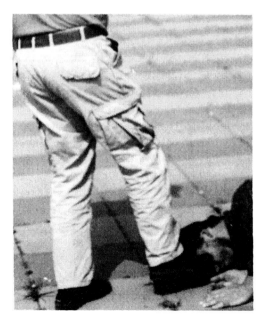

FOLLOW-UP KICK
TO THE HEAD.

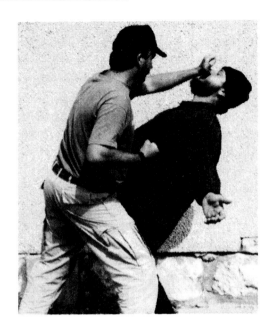

SMASH TO
THE NOSE.

you simultaneously throw the weight of your left shoulder behind the blow, striking upward with your elbow in the cocked and locked position. You want to smash into the area near the mouth so that the butt of your hand crashes up into the base of your enemy's nose. Don't be afraid to aim a little low, since the sliding motion of your hand will move you briskly to the target. What you don't want to do is aim high and miss. If you do this properly, your assailant's nose will shatter, plunging him into almost unbearable pain. If this blow is delivered with excess force, it will drive bone and cartilage up into the brain and result in death.

Follow-Up Blow

Almost immediately, swing your strong leg upward and smash your knee into your opponent's groin. That should settle accounts very nicely.

Note: The Adam's apple and nose targets are especially suited to women (or men) who don't have the physical capability needed for other moves. These targets only call for strong nerve, determination, and speed, not strength.

Battering Ram Blow

In the Mideast, a very popular variation for attacking your opponent's nose is using your own head as a weapon. For this type of attack, the heavy and well-boned head becomes a very formidable weapon when hurled against the relatively weak defenses of the human nose. This is a type of attack that is the least expected in the West, where it is almost unknown.

Crippling Blow

Jonathan told me he used this system in a recent altercation with extremely satisfying results. When your opponent moves toward you, grab his head in both hands, duck down slightly, and crash the front of your skull into his nose. He assures me that the human nose cracks like an eggshell, thus putting your adversary out of contention within seconds.

Follow-Up Blow

Jonathan favors a swift kick to the side of the knee joint, an area of extreme weakness for putting his opponent down for the count. This maneuver, if delivered sharply and accurately with the sole of the shoe, never fails to dislocate the knee—a very painful and yet nonlethal maneuver.

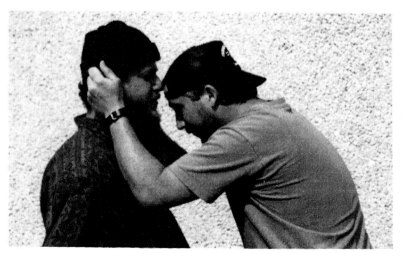

THE BATTERING RAM BLOW.

Boiler Room Blow

There are times when you are attacked and will not have the chance to deliver a fight-stopping Adam's apple or nose combo. Your enemy doesn't warn you but rather jumps you in the street. No better and softer target may present itself than your enemy's stomach. It's a big target and relatively easy to engage. The problem is that to do this properly you have to have much more strength than in all the preceding methods of taking an opponent out. This blow will do the trick but is much harder for the person of limited strength to deliver properly.

Crippling Blow

Step forward on your weak foot and deliver a blow with a closed fist smash directly into your enemy's gut somewhere below the belt line and in an upward direction. Deliver it with all of the strength you can muster and it should knock the wind out of him and leave him gasping for breath.

Follow-Up Blows

The chances are your assailant will be doubled over—a perfect opportunity to grab his hair with both hands, pulling

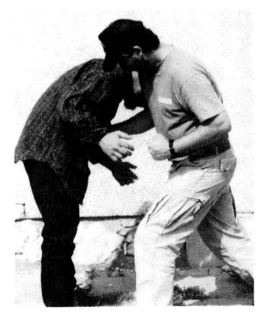

THE "BOILER ROOM" BLOW TO THE STOMACH.

his head down and forward while you smartly smash your strong knee up into his face. Do it more than once in a crisp series of moves, and he should be down and out. However, when he is down, use the opportunity to kick him in the head. Disgusting? Most assuredly. But also most effective.

STREET SURVIVAL LESSON

1) *Dirty fighting: the people's choice.* Dirty fighting is best suited for the average person who does not have the time, inclination, or skills needed to master the classical martial art disciplines.

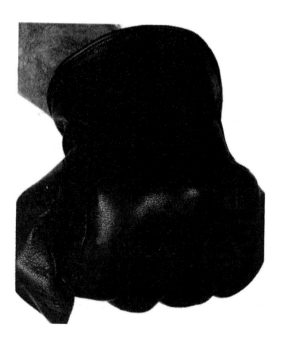

ENFORCING THE LAW: THE SP 99 Police Defender powdered lead tactical glove provides power to subdue perps when firearms are not called for.

HOUSEHOLD TOOL WEAPONS

A possible solution for those who are barred from carrying conventional weapons for self-defense is to substitute common household tools, such as monkey wrenches, hammers, and screwdrivers, for this task. These tools make quite formidable close-quarter weapons if one is forced to rely on them. The wrench and hammer become battle hammers, which can inflict quite deadly crushing blows. The screwdriver is a fair substitute for a puncturing knife blade or stiletto.

I would carry these items in a toolbox. If one is stopped in his car, one can certainly make a good case that the tools were for repair work needed in someone's home. Without going into details, suffice it to say this was being done by many Israelis during the earlier stages of the so-called Intifada.

GOLF CLUBS, BASEBALL BATS, CANES, UMBRELLAS

In the streets of New York, I noticed some individuals carrying golf clubs. While such "weapons" pass the criteria of appearing to be nonlethal, most of them have shanks that might not last more than one good blow to your adversary's head. On the other hand, if delivered with magnum force, one blow may prove more than adequate. Personally, I'd prefer the irons instead of the woods, for obvious reasons.

In general, golf clubs seem only suited to deliver crushing blows and are not the best choice for alternate weapon use. The extra reach they afford is wasted in the restricted number of blows they allow. They tend to be weak in the shank and thus a rather poor choice for self-defense.

I have picked up baseball bats on occasion when I saw trespassers on my land. The mere sight of such a potential weapon in hand usually results in such people taking off for parts unknown. However, I hasten to add the baseball bat was always backed up by a brace of .45 autos, just in case. Baseball bats are excellent for crushing blows. I have also found them excellent

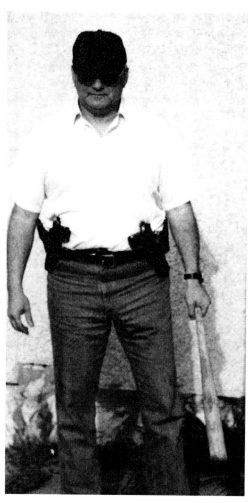

BASEBALL BAT ON THE JOB.

for warding off potential attackers while I reached for a pistol. Pointing one of these bats at them signals in a most primitive way that you mean business.

I have recently become enamored with canes when social circumstances dictate that solution (my gray hair blends in perfectly with them). There are two canes that can be highly recommended for street survival use. One is the Irish black thorn walking stick, which is light, extremely strong, and has the added effect of cutting your adversary, since the knots distributed along its shank present an uneven surface that punctures skin, muscle, and bone. A second choice is the very popular brass-headed hardwood cane. I've carried one of these on occasion but prefer the Irish black thorn. Incidentally, the natural hardwood head on the black thorn can deliver as good a crushing blow to your adversary's "noggin" as can the brass-headed portion of the hardwood cane, and the black thorn is definitely more controllable.

Targets selected for cane use should be those that maximize pain and crippling effect: the shin bone, ankle joint, and knee joint, as well as the corresponding parts of the human arm—the forearm, wrist, and elbow. Really good cane fighters can aim for the shoulder, neck, and temple. A strong blow to the neck or temple can easily kill an adversary.

GARDEN TOOL WEAPONS

Garden or agricultural tools have been used as weapons from time immemorial. The scythe, the sledgehammer, the shovel, the ax, the machete—all can be utilized for self-defense around the farm or home. They have always been the weapons of the peasants. They bring forth pictures in the mind of French farmers storming the Bastille or Mexican peasants in revolt.

Around the home or farm, such items are considered part of the landscape and will not even be noticed as potential weapons since they have ceased to be such for centuries. Nothing could be further from the truth. They can be quite formidable weapons of emergency—the sledgehammer and shovel for crushing, the ax for chopping, the scythe for slicing, and the machete for both.

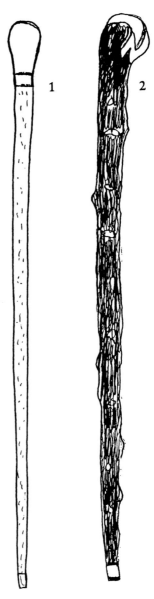

CANES: 1. Brass-headed hardwood; 2. Irish or English Blackthorn.

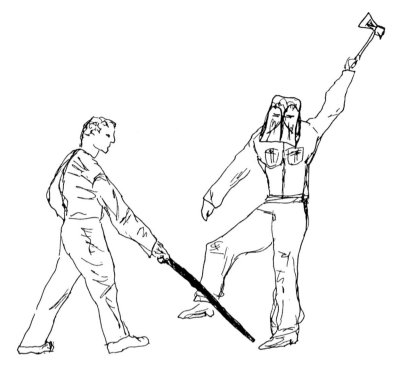

LOWER EXTREMITY CANE TARGETS: Inside of ankle, shinbone, knee.

CAR TOOLS

    Car repair tools such as tire irons (puncturing or crushing blows) and tire spanners (crushing blows) make another family of "nonweapon" weapons that can be used in a pinch or when necessitated by political madness or circumstance. The host of ever-increasing antigun laws around the globe, some of which are already in existence, make thinking about the use of such alternate weapons practical.

STREET SURVIVAL LESSONS

1)   *Be inventive!* See all objects around you with an eye

toward weapon use. Tools especially lend themselves to being utilized in an emergency as lethal weapons.

2) *Know your history.* If you remember your history, you will recall that most items found around a farm or home were once used as close-quarter weapons, not only by individuals but by armies of men.

3) *Blows by substitute weaponry.* Everyday items can be used to deliver the following blows, either singly or in combination: crushing blows, slicing blows, stabbing blows.

4) *Your opponent can be inventive.* Be aware of this fact. He may choose an item that at first glance looks quite harmless but can be used with deadly effect.

....

BLADED WEAPONS OF COLD IRON

Gold is for the mistress—silver for the maid
Copper for the craftsman cunning in his trade.
"Good!" said the Baron, sitting in his hall
But iron—cold iron—is master of them all.

—Rudyard Kipling

Bladed weapons are the most common weapons in use around the world and range from pen knives to machetes. Swords have mostly fallen by the wayside in the West, but personally, if I were restricted to defending my life with a bladed weapon, I would unhesitatingly pick a good sword, emphasis being on the word good, since the chance of finding a well-made sword blade today is quite difficult. Swords are seen here on Israel television, used by the PLO and HAMAB to dispatch Arabs deemed enemies to paradise—more than 1,000 in the current Intifada alone. They have also been seen in riots and were used in the Arab uprisings of 1929, 1936–39, and 1948 to murder Jews who had the misfortune of falling into Arab hands.

The Machete

The machete could be labeled the "poor man's sword." I've seen quite respectable examples made right at home, though very low-cost models can be purchased in many hardware and gun stores. It's the peasant's sword of Latin America.

The machete is an agricultural tool that has been designed primarily for cutting grass and crops. This would be akin to slashing or chopping in a fight. It accomplishes this task extremely well. It is, however, much slower than, say, a fine Bowie knife with a 9- to 10-inch blade in a classical knife fight, knife against knife.

The Ax

Axes, like knives, come in all sizes and shapes, from small camp axes to lumber axes. Axes have been the chosen bladed weapon of Mideast terrorists, since they are well-designed for chopping up their victims. Mutilation and dismemberment are the norm for them. Axes do not make good fighting weapons unless accompanied by a stout shield held in your weak hand to ward off any counterattacks by your assailant. If your adversary is forewarned and is armed with a bowie or machete, the ax wielder can only chop at his enemy, and to do this he must raise his arm, thus exposing his body to swift and deadly counterattack. The shield he carries into battle protects the ax fighter from such a counterattack to this most vital part of his anatomy.

The Bowie

I consider the bowie knife the best classical fighting knife ever designed. We must remember that by the word classical, we are speaking of a knife fight between two opponents that takes place in an area that is called the circle of death. Such deadly confrontations are a rarity today but can and do occur. A good bowie with a 9- to 10-inch blade is the perfect

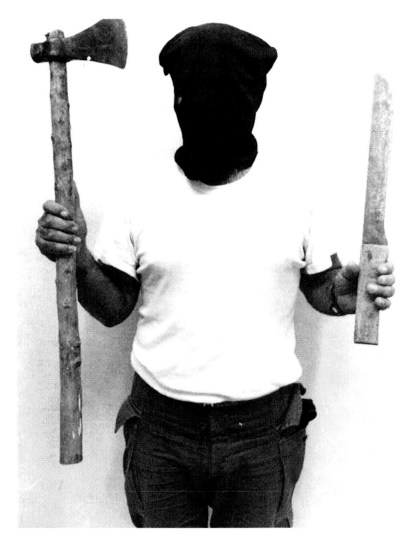

TERRORIST IN UNIFORM: The hood, ax, and knife.

weapon for such a fight. With such a bowie, you can slash, stab, and, most importantly, chop your adversary in an efficient manner.

This said, the problem with the bowie remains that it is big . . . very big. I know men who carry them, but when I check the blades, I invariably find that they have been reduced to the 5- to 7-inch length. These midget bowies may look like bowies, but those carrying them may be fooling themselves. I am not partial to short-bladed bowie impostors. I feel you might as well get a good double-edged fighting knife such as the Applegate-Fairbairn Double-Edged Fighting Knife, which is far superior.

The bowie only makes sense when it can utilize the chopping blow along with the stab and slash, and to do this efficiently, you need weight and leverage, hence the long 9- to 10-inch blade. The problem is, such a classic bowie usually proves much too large as a practical street-carry knife unless one uses it as a primary weapon or as a back-up to a single handgun. Since I carry a brace of handguns and eight magazines, I carry the 9- to 10-inch bowie less and less, as it does seem overly large. I am much happier with my Applegate-Fairbairn Double-Edged Fighting Knife, which fills the bill as far as human engineering and fighting ability are concerned.

For people who can afford it, I would recommend a Bagwell Bowie. Bagwell and a handful of custom knife makers like him know what heat treatment of steel is all about. Purchasing such a knife is really purchasing a family heirloom—something to be passed from generation to generation with pride. For factory bowies, I would go to Cold Steel or Randall. I have a Cold Steel Trailmaster bowie and have never regretted buying it. It is a top-quality factory knife. I also had a Randall bowie, and the knife was equally special. The rule is, make sure you buy from people who take pride in their work and know what quality blades and knife making are all about. Anything else is a gamble. You may get lucky, and then again, you may have your blade fail you out there in the street at a most inopportune moment. That is a calamity to be avoided at all costs, especially if your knife is your primary weapon. Choose your blades for street carry very carefully. Looks alone won't do.

Case Study: Cutting Up with a Bowie

I live along the highway to Jerusalem in a section of the

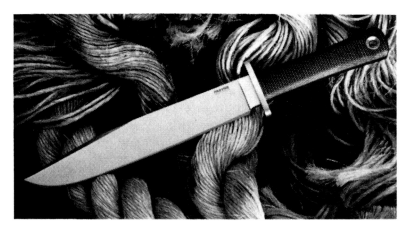

COLD STEEL TRAILMASTER BOWIE: Its upper false edge should be sharpened for the street. An excellent factory bowie with ample length (9 1/2 inches) and weight (22 ounces) for chopping. Fast and deadly.

country called the Judean Hills. It's heavily forested with pine trees. About a half mile from my house, I have a very large coop that can be used for egg-laying chickens. I have decided not to bother with this and instead have rented the empty coop to a fellow who is in the used cardboard box business. At times the coop is filled with as many as 50,000 of these things, making it a potential fire hazard.

Nomads coming over the hills from nearby villages that are not noted for their friendliness to people of my ilk work in the area. When the noonday heat and sun become too much, they enjoy camping with their sheep in the shade. Unfortunately, they especially enjoy the shade afforded by my coop and like to light fires to brew their Turkish coffee.

No matter how many times I asked in a most genteel manner, they continued to do this, turning the whole area into a disaster waiting to happen. It got so bad they even pitched a tent and made an area to tie their donkeys up in. Reasoning with them seemed to do me no good, as they obviously mistook my gentlemanly manner as a sign of weakness (unfortunately a very common error of certain ethnic groups in the Mideast when they meet North Americans).

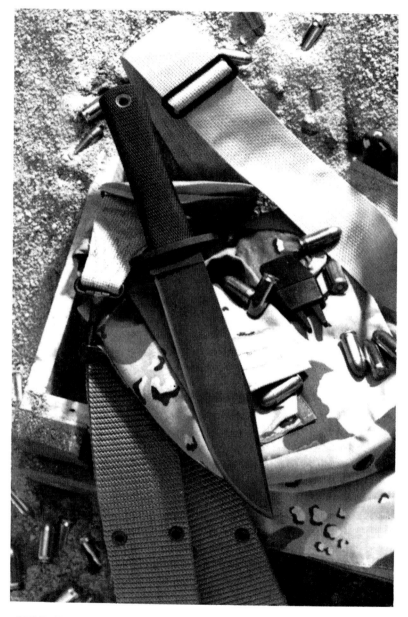

COLD STEEL RECON SCOUT: *A quality bowie, but with a 7 1/2-inch blade that offers increased portability at the cost of less chopping efficiency.*

One afternoon, I was returning to my home and noticed that they had not taken their tent down. I was faced with a clear choice—remove it, or as certain as light follows night it would soon be replaced with a tin hut and then finally a cinder block building from which they would then claim squatter's rights.

Dropping my wife off at home, I assured her that to do nothing would probably have them making coffee in her kitchen within the year. I proceeded to drive down to the coop and exit the car, Louisville Slugger baseball bat in my left hand, right hand free to get my Armond Swenson-Colt 1911, loaded with Hydro-Shoks and Black Talons and sitting in my Bianchi #50 Chapman Hi-Ride in the front cross-draw position under my jacket. Another 1911 rested on my strong-side hip.

As is usual in such confrontations in this part of the world, I was greeted with Salaams from three men who jumped up smiling and offered me black Turkish coffee they had just brewed. I stood in silence. When they saw the look on my face, they backed off.

Drawing my Cold Steel Trailmaster bowie from under my shirt, I quietly proceeded to cut the tent ropes and ropes that tethered their donkeys, chasing them off in the bargain. Within minutes, the tent was cut up into large doilies. This was done with a certain panache that convinced the squatters it was the better part of wisdom to leave this crazy Westerner alone.

I share this story with you as an example of the field use of the Trailmaster bowie—a bizarre test that it probably was never put to before. I can attest that everything they say about this knife is true; it definitely cuts rope.

The Double-Edged Fighting Knife

Double-edged fighting knives such as the Randall #2, the Kershaw Trooper, the Al Mar Shadow, the Gerber Mark 1 and 2, the Applegate-Fairbairn, and so on are among the most popular carry-knife designs for fighting ever designed. One of their big attributes is that you will actually carry them. They are handier than that big bowie you have up on the wall.

Probably the best-designed double-edged fighting knife in the world today is the Applegate-Fairbairn. Its factory version is manufactured by Blackjack Knives, Ltd. While I have been told by some that it's an improved Fairbairn-Sykes Commando Dagger, the improvements are so far-reaching and thought out as to make the comparison meaningless. It's like comparing a good Model T to an excellent new Rolls Royce. The improved design is the work of Col. Rex Applegate, former associate of W.E. Fairbairn and now dean of modern knife-fighting techniques as well as the world-renowned authority on close-quarter combat. His works are many. His book *Kill or Get Killed* is the classic on the subject (not to mention some of his other works, such as *Riot Control* and *Scouting and Patrolling,* basic texts on these subjects that are also available from Paladin Press).

For a combat knife that is ideally suited for its task, I prefer the double-edged Applegate-Fairbairn, which is well-balanced, fast, easy to carry, and superbly suited for its primary use, close-quarter fighting.

The Exotics

I like exotic knives. They look nice up on the wall. When well made, they are a pleasure to behold. If poorly made, as most are, I consider them an abomination. But one thing they are not. In my opinion they are not the best choice of fighting knives.

The wavy-bladed Indonesian *kris*, the *kard* Persian dagger, the Arab *jambiya*, the Gurkha *kukri*, the Indian *katar*, the Turkish *bichag*—all have been bloodied in battle, but all are inferior to a real bowie or a good double-edged fighting knife. Many are over-specialized. A good example is the *kukri*, a knife that the Gurkhas carry and use in battle not to fight with but rather to decapitate their enemies. It's more of a glorified ax than a fighting knife. After all, creeping up on your enemy and chopping his head off is not a knife fight, it is an ambush.

As for me, I'll leave those exotics up on the wall along with other artifacts. Use them as a first choice in a real knife fight? Never. Let my enemies carry them.

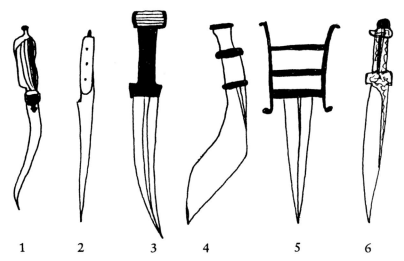

EXOTIC KNIVES: *1. Indonesian kris; 2. kard Persian dagger; 3. Arab jambiya; 4. Ghurka kukri; 5. Indian katar; 6. Turkish bichag.*

Boot Knives

While still called concealed fighting knives, many of today's designs have gone too far and are only minimal defense knives of miscellaneous design. They can be double-edged or single-edged, "trick" designs in belt buckles, push daggers, tiny daggers, "open pocket knives," skeleton knives, etc. The major design trend is aimed at minimizing and miniaturizing knives to look like serious fighters while eliminating any chance of their actually doing this task with any degree of efficiency.

Short-bladed boot knives (less than 4 inches) do have the good attribute of being at hand in an emergency, and many people believe in them. The problem is, many of them are really only suited for stabbing and not much else. In the hands of someone who has taken the time to study human anatomy, they may suffice. But in the hands of an amateur who is only posturing, they can get one killed, since simply stabbing an adversary at random with one of these may not do the trick.

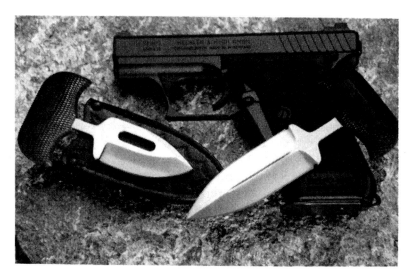

COLD STEEL DEFENDER BOOT KNIVES: Such push design boot knives are at their best as weapons of ambush.

The whole question of what is legal blade length, etc., is probably the main reason for the popularity of such knives.

Of course, anyone wanting to carry "legal" in some jurisdictions is likely to choose something that at least resembles what he really would like to carry in its big brother form. A host of confusing antiknife laws has spawned the confusion and variety of designs that we call boot knives today.

Pocket Folders

Pocket knives are probably the most common form of knife carried in the street, ranging from tiny 1-inch bladed utility knives to 4-inch folding (and camouflaged as such) fighters.

This type of knife, along with the boot knife, has grown in popularity for self-defense use because of the multitude of antiknife laws that have sprung up in many areas of the world. These laws include most sheath knives and pocket knives with long blades. The usual 4 inches seems to be the cut-off point for legal folding blades in the street. The reason for this is the fact that 4 inches is the usual length considered legal in the United States, and most nations take their guidelines from America.

The jackknives or folding hunters have one problem in common: they take time to open, and most require two hands to complete this task. Much improvement in design has allowed some models to be opened with one hand and still not fall into the category of that most feared and highly overrated knife of Hollywood films, the switchblade. When purchasing such a knife, buy a quality name brand, since if used for self-defense, the blades of the cheaper ones will typically break or their locking mechanisms will fail when bone is struck. Under this unfortunate circumstance, the blade will then fold back, slicing finger tendons and blood vessels and instantly crippling your strong hand, setting you up for the coup de grace.

For this reason, too, I do not recommend any folding knife that is not of a lock-back design for anything but household tasks.

Lock-Back Folders

Good utility folders that can double as fighting knives in a pinch are those made by Buck, Gerber, Cold Steel, and Spiderco. While certainly not the first choice of fighting knife by anyone even slightly trained in the subject, they can and do fill a niche created by bureaucrats bent on disarming the honest public. When wanting a hideout knife that does not raise the eyebrows of those looking for such items, the lock-back folder design of pocket knives fills the bill quite nicely.

The Spiderco Police Model is an excellent example of the genre. What is good about the design is that it is very easy to carry and conceal since it incorporates a clip that holds the knife to the trouser top, shirt, edge of the pocket, etc. It does this so comfortably that one can almost forget it's there. The serrated blade model works just like they claim—excellent for cutting seat belts in case of a car accident. The standard edge is an excellent slicer. The truth is I own a pair and carry

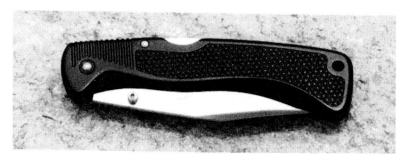

COLD STEEL VOYAGER. A one-piece Zytel lock-back knife that is ultralight (3.3 ounces), strong, and sports a 4-inch blade.

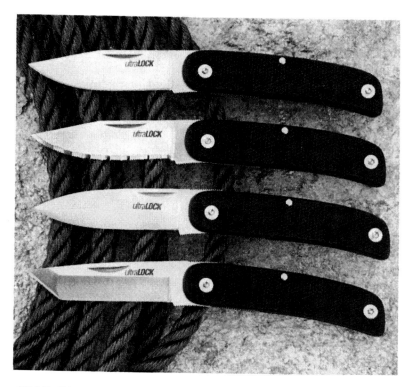

COLD STEEL ULTRALOCKS (left to right): Clip, serrated, spear, and tanto points.

them both on occasion. I also have a good Buck folder with a
Damascus blade and horn grips, as well as a Puma stainless-
steel bladed model. All do quite well as hideout weapons that
still look relatively harmless. They do fill in the gap between
a good bowie or an Applegate-Fairbairn Double-Edged
Fighter and the smaller vest-pocket or boot knives. They
accomplish a multitude of useful tasks and, because of this,
are becoming the knives most often chosen for the street.

The Balisong

I do not much like the *balisong* knife from the
Phillippines, believing its hinge joint is a most likely place for
structural failure to occur if bone is hit. To date, I have not
inspected any model that causes me to change this negative
opinion. I believe the design has a lot of writer's hype behind
it. It's a lot of sizzle and very little steak. While a whole
school of supposedly proven street-fighting technique is built
around the *balisong* design, I believe that much better knife

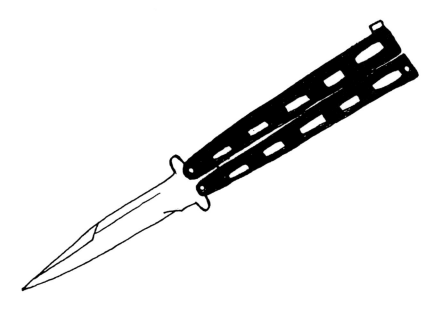

BALISONG: The hinge joint is the weak part of this design.

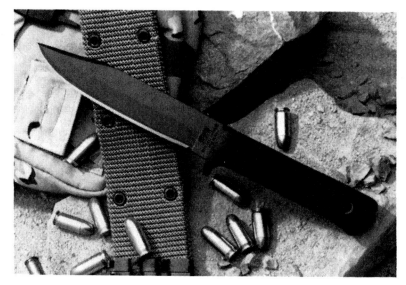

COLD STEEL SRK: A survival/rescue knife with a tough 6-inch blade that is well-suited to the primary task it was designed for.

designs are on the market. It is sort of the derringer of knives—dreams, exotic ideas that may fail in the cold reality of the street.

Beware of Junk Knives

This is a very large category of knives that spans the entire spectrum from fair quality to atrocious. Blade size and shape vary as much as quality.

Some of those formidable looking knives I've seen around in gun stores leave me cold. For example, I can see no use in having those heavy serrations on the spine portion of knife blades, since in every test I've ever conducted, they have failed to perform as promised. I've come to the conclusion that if you have need of a saw, buy a saw and leave the more mundane utility chores or fighting uses to the knife. This is true except in one case. If you are a pilot of a light plane or copter, these formidable looking serrations may be useful (again, only in a strong, quality blade) to cut through the

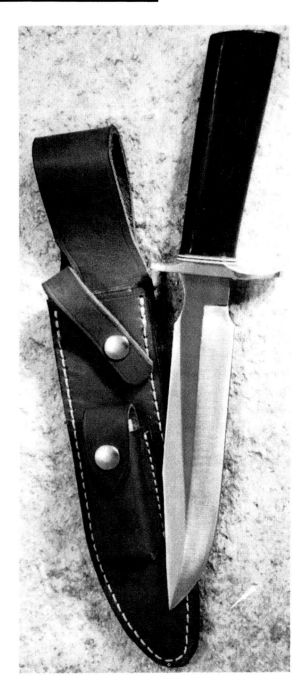

COLD STEEL RI
MILITARY
CLASSIC:
A quality 7-inch
blade.

very thin aluminum skin of aircraft. This is the only case where they may do the job they are intended to do, but once again, this is only in a quality blade and not one of those junk blades that have no proper heat treatment applied to them by skilled knifesmiths. Cheap knives will snap or bend under hard use, and cutting yourself out of an airplane (for those envisioning such uses) is not what one would call an easy task.

A good knife blade, especially a fighting knife, should have a point that will not snap and an edge that will stay sharp even after hard use. Most of the knives around that I have seen are fairly good lookers but poor performers.

No Bargain

I remember being in New York City a few years back and seeing a street vendor selling stainless-steel knives sporting 6-inch bowie-type blades with serrated spines. They were hollow-handled and had compasses in the rear of their grips. Now hollow-handled knives are another one of those "dream weapons" of Hollywood that can turn into a nightmare out on the street. They are extremely difficult to make properly, and many times their blades are not supported firmly enough for serious use. As I inspected the knife, I realized the Asian manufacturer had given the buyer just about everything the buyer demanded except quality. Why, it even had a sheath with a sharpening stone in it.

I asked, "How much?"

"One buck," he replied. What a bargain.

How could anyone go wrong for a buck? So for fun, I plunked down my buck and took my chances.

When I got back to the farm, I put it into the large metal box that I keep my dog food in, planning to use it to open the thick plastic bags that hold my dog's commercial dog food. After using it on those tough bags, I can report that I got screwed out of a buck. Both knife blade and serrations were consistently defeated by those plastic bags. Never buy looks or low cost.

STREET SURVIVAL LESSONS

1) *The sword is king.* The most effective bladed weapon is a good sword.

2) *Machete—the poor man's sword.* While labeled as such, the machete can be quite unwieldy. It is really a slash-and-chop weapon of stealth.

3) *The ax—king of the choppers.* Beware of choosing an ax unless you use a shield. The ax is the supreme weapon of stealth, but a poor fighter when used alone.

4) *Bowie—classical fighting knife.* The bowie is ideally suited for the classic circle of death in the ideal 9- to 10-inch blade length. A shorter blade will have no chopping efficiency, and a longer one (11 inches or more) is too slow. It's usually too heavy for daily street carry, unless you use it as your primary arm or in some cases as a back-up weapon to a handgun.

5) *The double-edged fighting knife.* These are the best knives if you want a fast, easily controlled fighting knife that you will have on you at all times. As a tertiary weapon, the 6-inch blade is best (when legal, of course). Beware of those very long blade designs like the Arkansas toothpick (9- to 14-inch blades). They never will surpass a good 9- to 10-inch bowie

6) *Beware: exotic knives.* Most exotic knives are really not suited for modern knife fighting. Many are made of poor steel and will fail at the critical moment. Many are poorly designed and suited only for one task. These are lookers, not fighters.

7) *Caution: boot knives.* Most boot knives made today are really only miniaturized copies of more serious knives. Many are over-designed to the point that they fulfill a role only in the mind of the person carrying them and will fail out in the real world. If you carry a boot knife, make it a serious full-sized design. If this is legally impossible, then know its very real limitations in serious street combat.

8) *Pocket folders.* Standard pocket folders are utility knives that may be used for self-defense. However, they are almost always a poor choice, since they tend to easily break their locks or fold back at the least amount of force applied to them.

9) *Lock-back folders.* A good lock-back folder is a knife whose time may have come. They can be of legal size, made to open easily with one hand, and, if a quality design, will be sufficiently strong to be used in a knife fight.

10) *Beware: the balisong.* The lockwork on these knives, unless they are of very good construction, may tend to break if heavy bone or muscle is struck. These are more in the line of slashing knives.

11) *Buy quality.* As in all things, buy quality. This is especially true with knives, since a well finished but inferior knife can fool you into thinking you have something good. This can even be true of higher-priced hollow-handled knives that are nicely polished and finished and have huge blades or spines of formidable serrations that don't saw. They will snap like peanut brittle if put to the test. Price has nothing to do with quality. They can all fail, just as surely as that fun junker I bought in New York at a buck a throw.

AMBUSH AND ASSASSINATION VS. A KNIFE FIGHT

If you have the grave misfortune of being caught unaware by a street punk bent on doing you in, you are in deep trouble. For ambush or assassination almost any weapon will do, and a good case can be made for so-called cold weapons since they have the advantage of being silent, thus allowing your assailant to do the deed and then slip away unnoticed.

For this type of attack, even a lady's hat pin stuck into a vital part of the human brain will cause death. The weapon becomes secondary to stealth and execution of the act itself. The secret of surviving ambush-type attacks where almost everything favors your opponent is eternal alertness. Don't get into that situation. Remember the alley cat.

I am presently teaching Israeli settlers these facts of life, since they (along with the rest of us Israelis) face ambush and assassination as a daily and routine part of life. This applies to women and children and not only to the soldier or police officer. Predators do not differentiate much when committing murder. Ambush and assassination have nothing to do with knife fighting, yet the two are often mixed up in the minds of people who should know better.

It must be remembered that the purpose of a true knife fight is not to jump your opponent and slit his throat. That would not be a knife fight; that would be assassination. The true knife fighter knows that the chances of killing his forewarned and armed opponent immediately in a sudden attack is highly unlikely, and that this tactic is very dangerous if foiled. Rather, he chooses the path of a sort of mini war of attrition based on a strategic plan of first crippling his adversary, neutralizing his ability to fight back, and finally ending it by delivering the coup de grace.

The goal of a true knife fight that takes place in the arena called the circle of death is to slowly slice and whittle down an opponent so that his defenses are breached, all the time keeping damage to oneself to zero or at least a minimum. It's a matter of who loses the most blood first, who becomes

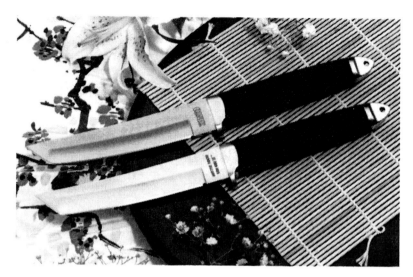

COLD STEEL TANTOS: Excellent for piercing and cross-slashing in a knife fight, but handicapped by a lack of backslash and chopping capabilities. Best as knives of stealth.

more and more immobile, and who weakens the fastest. It is a war of attrition.

If you want to become a formidable street knife fighter, you have to study human anatomy. You should be very aware of all the target areas and well-versed in the feinting, slashing, stabbing, and chopping techniques needed to disable them.

This must be done in an instinctive, unconscious manner, as spoken about in the chapter on the correct mind-set. It is not easy. It is bloody and brutal. This may be why the true classic knife fighter is such a rarity today.

THE CIRCLE OF DEATH: THE CLASSICAL KNIFE FIGHT

Unlike ambush and assassination, knife fighting takes place between two armed and aware opponents. Classical knife fighting is a very bloody, messy, and dangerous business. But then again, so is life itself. Joe, a friend of mine, likes to say, "Life is very dangerous, you know. I never heard of anyone getting out of it alive." In classical knife fighting, we could say, "A true knife fight between two somewhat evenly matched and well-armed opponents is very dangerous. They will probably be slashed, stabbed, and chopped up—winner and loser both."

Only a few days ago, such a knife fight was reported on Israel TV. It seems that two recent Jewish immigrants from Ethiopia, both young men, had some quarrel and decided to pull their knives and settle it out in the street. In the end, both bled to death from their wounds.

Sharpened, bladed weapons have been with us even since the Stone Age, when primitive man first learned to sharpen hard flint into a weapon. Since then, bladed weapons have been improved and designed to continue to do this task. No culture on earth, no matter how advanced or primitive, has put aside the sharpened weapon.

In ancient Egypt, the copper dagger was used. With the Hittites, we saw the first true iron blade, a weapon that has been improved upon constantly to this, the age of space rockets and computers. It is therefore easy to predict that bladed weapons will be around in one form or another even when we carry laser weapons for street survival. The blade remains one of the most fearsome and deadly forms of weapon ever revised by the hand and brain of homo sapiens.

A well-honed cold iron blade is one of the fastest and most efficient means of dispatching an enemy. It stabs, slashes, and sometimes even chops an adversary to ribbons, releasing buckets of blood in the process. Far messier than a gunshot wound, a knife wound isn't what you'd call a lovely sight to behold. Ask any emergency ward orderly in a major American city on a Saturday night, who works in an environment that resembles a slaughterhouse.

Bladed weapons are very popular with street punks or terrorists because of their lower cost and availability. They remain popular because they are an extremely handy and silent means of dispatching an unsuspecting victim.

Correct Mind-Set in the Circle of Death

Because close-quarter knife fighting is so bloody and deadly, it requires nerves of steel. Victory belongs to the swift and aggressive who, finding themselves in the circle of death—a radius of a meter or two—facing another knife-wielding antagonist, stay cool in what is probably one of the scariest combat experiences known to man. Cultures that stress bladed weapons respect them, for they know the damage they do. I have a friend who worked against Islamic terrorists in Lebanon, and he told me they were more intimidated by the large bowie knife in his belt than by his S&W Model 645 auto and his M16 rifle. There must be something to the fear of castration theory, which is unfortunately not a theory if you have the misfortune of falling into their bloody hands.

Handling Fear

If you are accosted in the street and find yourself in a knife fight, you will most likely feel an overpowering sense of fear. It is almost certain that your opponent will be experiencing the same fear, though he may mask it behind a shield of bravado.

Don't be ashamed of reasonable fear. Does everyone feel it? Possibily not to the same degree. There are those "fighters" again. But even they would admit to feeling at least uneasy in such a situation. The most important thing about fear is how you treat it. To control and use it to your advantage is the goal. Turn it into disciplined anger. Get mad. That S.O.B. wants to slice you up. That should enrage you! Turn the tables on your attacker and do unto him what he wants to do unto you. Controlled anger and an explosive counterattack will swing the initiative to you and act as a first step toward your dominating the circle of death.

The knife, like any weapon, can act as a deterrent, its mere presence signaling to your potential opponent that he will have to pay a high price if he engages you in the street. Once again, the key is your mental attitude. Your opponent must believe that you are serious and will fight to the death, using the knife as a means of dispatching him to hell. But remember, if you do decide to fight and not use flight, make sure you aren't bluffing yourself. Pulling a knife and then deciding it's all just a bluff is a sure way of getting yourself killed if the bluff doesn't work.

Remember, knife cultures do exist around the world. Your opponent may come from such a culture. He may be well-versed in such combat and have the scars to prove it. Never bluff with any weapon. Whatever you do, be prepared to carry it out to the bitter end. A close-quarter knife fight usually can't be broken off, as drawn blood only encourages its continuation.

Basic Knife Motions

The Slash: Cross and Back. This is a sweeping motion that slices across your opponent's anatomy. The slash can be executed in a forward (cross) or backward motion (back slash), which usually follows the forward slash. The purpose of the slash is to open up a series of bleeding cuts and sever tendons. It is used in wearing down your opponent. On occasion, the slash may cut a vital artery and thus can end a knife

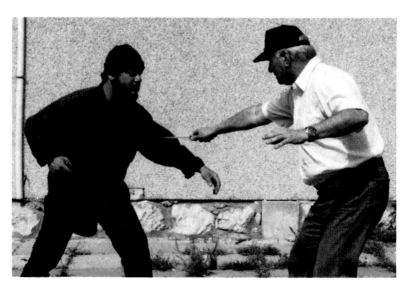

THE CROSS SLASH.

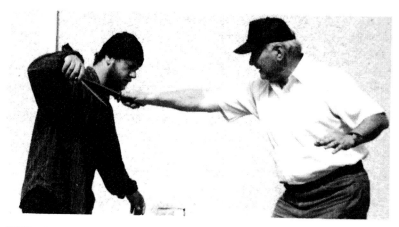

THE BACK SLASH. A target of opportunity—your adversary's knife hand.

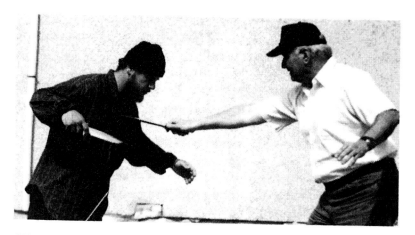

THE HORIZONTAL THRUST.

fight quickly. It can be used to feint (fake an opponent out). Slashing, the safest offensive tactic employed in a knife fight, is favored by all professionals.

The Stab: Overhead. The overhead stab so favored in novels and films is the mark of the amateur (as is throwing the knife from hand to hand) and is supposedly a sure sign that you've lucked out in a knife fight.

But is that really true? How can anyone in a knife fight

consider the circumstances he faces lucky for him? Sure, the books and magazines say you're lucky to face a stabber, but could they be wrong? Maybe your adversary is a pro who is faking you out, making you think he doesn't know much about knife fighting. While the overhead stab leaves one wide open for counterattack and should be avoided like the plague, the use of it by your opponent may be a bluff. Most important of all, even if it is not a bluff, the knife wielder is still very dangerous, especially if he uses an explosive, aggressive attack. Never get too self-confident under an uplifted blade. No one holding a sharp blade is that easy to defeat. Even rank amateurs have been known to win lethal confrontations.

The Stab (Thrust): Horizontal. The stab used in a thrusting motion does have its place in a knife fight and is especially useful when feinting. It can also be very useful if you spot an opening in your opponent's defensives that allows its safe, effective use. However, it is still only an adjunct to the slash unless your opponent is disabled and you use it to finish him off. Another time is when you have fended off your opponent's attack and are going into a counterattack. However, such a move puts you into your opponent's strike zone and makes you very vulnerable. Use the thrust with supreme caution.

The Chop. The use of a strong chopping blow to sever bone and muscle necessitates the carrying of a knife designed to do this. The very best design for this extra capability is the bowie with a blade of 9 to 10 inches, since it does not sacrifice speed and can still deliver a strong chopping blow. It has the weight and strength needed, which is the reason it remains the king of all classic circle of death knives. Jim Bowie knew what he needed when he designed his knife.

Most fighting knives do not have the capability of severing an arm or hand. They lack the weight and blade length for proper leverage. There are some exceptions, like the *kukri* knife, but all it can really do is chop. It is not a fighting knife but a weapon of ambush and assassination used to split or decapitate an enemy's skull. In that, it resembles a very light battle-ax.

Knives for the Circle of Death

It is my opinion that only two knife designs fit the bill for the circle of death. While I like the bowie with a 9- to 10-inch blade, I find it too cumbersome when wearing a brace of .45s to make it worthwhile. That is why I and so many others find the Applegate-Fairbairn Double-Edged Fighting Knife so practical. With it one can engage in all sorts of tasks, not the least of which is the silent killing of one's adversary. True, it does not chop off limbs, but unless you find yourself in a classical knife fight and you are up against a 9-inch bowie wielded by someone who knows how to use it in such a manner, this is no serious disadvantage. The Double-Edged Fighting Knife is portable and fast, and chances are you'll have it on you and not on the wall at home.

Again, avoid exotic blades such as *kukris, kris,* or even trench knives, bayonets, or OSS-type daggers. These are weapons of assassination that make poor fighting knives. If

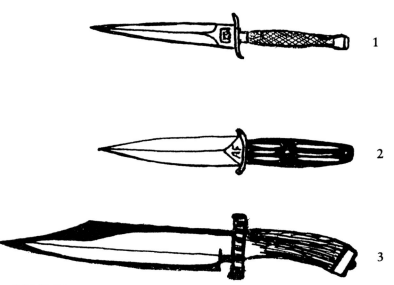

COMBAT KNIFE TRIO: 1. Fairbairn-Sykes Commando Knife, a thrusting design; 2. Applegate-Fairbairn Double-Edged Fighting Knife, capable of thrusting and slashing; 3. Bowie with 9- to 10-inch blade, capable of thrusting, slashing, and chopping but handicapped by its size.

pressed, I would prefer a good folding hunter to many of these types. Your fighting knife should have a good heft and feel in the hand, fitting comfortably so that you can take a firm grip.

Never Throw Your Knife Away

Another canard is the hero throwing his knife at his adversary—sheer nonsense, since the chance of penetrating a vital spot on your antagonist's anatomy with sufficient force is next to zero. Add to this the fact that you have disarmed yourself and armed your enemy, making you a candidate for not only fool of the year but death.

Real knife fighting consists of a series of forward and backward slashing cuts executed with a strong and razor-sharp blade. That is why the bowie or a double-edged fighting knife blade design is needed. They allow you to slice your opponent in the forward or backward slash without rotating your wrist. Of course, a very keen cutting edge is critical or you won't get the desired result.

All knives must have a good sheath to protect the blade and a good whetstone-type sharpener to keep said blade keen. These items must also be of the highest quality.

FAIRBAIRN'S SIX PRIMARY TARGETS

During World War II, Maj. W.E. Fairbairn, codesigner of the famed commando knife along with Sykes, accumulated actual documented evidence of combat use of knives and ascertained that every knife fighter must keep his enemy's primary targets in mind so as to better cut into these critical life-supporting areas. Fairbairn picked areas of the body he deemed accessible in a knife fight. Some experts disagree with some of his choices, but all agree his vision of primary targets was sound.

The Heart

The problem with the heart is that it is encased behind heavy bone and muscle, and only a thrust of considerable

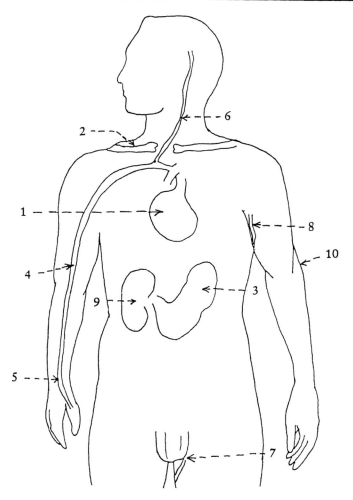

BLADED WEAPON TARGETS: 1. heart, 2. subclavian artery,
3. stomach, 4. brachial artery, 5. radial artery, 6. carotid artery,
7. femoral artery, 8. auxiliary artery, 9. kidney.

force can put it out of operation. The fact that it is behind the breastbone or heavy ribs and is protected by inches of hard muscle make it an extremely difficult target to even reach. Also, there is a danger that your knife will actually lodge in this protective shield and necessitate your using two hands to pull it out, a very dicey tactic in close-quarter combat. Deep stab wounds have the unfortunate tendency to contract around what is penetrating the body, grasping the projectile in a vacuumlike vise.

A more serious problem is the necessity of having to strike directly at the heart in a thrust that opens you up to swift counterattack. Some say to save the heart stab for when your opponent is down, waiting for the fatal coup de grace.

The Subclavian Artery

This artery is hidden behind the so-called collarbone, and because of this is extremely difficult to reach with any degree of certainty. This is a target for the expert who can handle the task of breaching its defenses.

The Stomach

The stomach is an excellent candidate for slashing cuts being easily breached by a razor-sharp blade. Many experts believe the abdominal artery, located some 4 to 6 inches under the skin, is also a good target, but this is a false assumption. To get to this blood vessel requires a deep, stabbing thrust, which should be followed immediately by a slashing, ripping motion across the area. Not a recommended procedure in a fast-moving close-quarter knife fight, since your opponent could use the time to complete his attack while you are so dangerously exposed. Stick with the stomach; it is an excellent, easily ruined target of opportunity that is large in size and near the surface of the skin.

The Brachial Artery

This is a more easily attacked artery that is located in the upper arm and is usually exposed in a knife fight as your adversary moves his knife at you. Remember, both arms have such an artery, and both are therefore good candidates for attack. Experienced street fighters like to slash this artery across the inner arm and directly above the elbow. They use a feinting motion, followed by a slash. Like all arteries, this artery, if completely severed, will result in loss of consciousness in about 60 seconds, followed by almost immediate death. The brachial artery is a very important target and should be a major goal in any knife fight.

The Radial Artery

This artery runs across the top of the forearm, follows the radius bone (a bone in line with the thumb), and branches off in a few directions, such as the elbow joint, the wrist, the thumb, and finally to the index finger. During its trek, it is covered by a host of tendons and nerves, inviting easy accessibility to disabling cuts. Any cut on your opponent's knife-holding arm will most likely force him to drop the weapon, making him a sitting duck in a fight.

In a street fight, it is important to remember the radial is closest to the surface along the wrist, making this area a very high priority for attack. Actually, in a knife fight, your opponent's forearm is a most vulnerable target and should be attacked vigorously with constant effort. It should be engaged by first using a proper feint followed by a slash.

The Carotid Artery

In close proximity to the jugular vein, the carotid artery runs along the side of the neck and is associated with vital brain functions as well as the windpipe. It should be considered a very important target to be attacked with a series of well-executed feints followed up with a forward or backward slash, or even a thrust, since it is very accessible. Severing this artery ends the fight and your opponent's life in seconds.

In attacking this artery, one must keep in mind that even missing it completely may end the fight since the neck is so filled with vital parts—for example, the larynx (Adam's apple) and the trachea (windpipe)—that a slash to the area can result in shock death.

SURPRISE TARGETS OF OPPORTUNITY

After the six targets listed by Major Fairbairn, some of

which everyone agrees with and some (like the heart) that are controversial, we have what we call targets of opportunity. In the circle of death, it must be constantly kept in mind that any cut, no matter how seemingly insignificant, weakens your opponent both mentally and physically. Sting him anywhere, for even a slight jab may put his mind off balance and cause him to concentrate on the hurt and not on you. Maybe the cut is nonlethal, but it will confuse and intimidate your adversary and, if delivered properly, might even disorient him and induce temporary shock. When and if this occurs, attack! You must capitalize on every opportunity by delivering a series of feints, thrusts, slashes, and chops so that the initiative stays with you or is moved toward you as you work your way toward his throat, the ultimate target of opportunity. He who dominates a knife fight wins.

Use Surprise
All through the Bible, the Hebrews won against far superior odds by using the element of surprise. This tactic is still used today in modern Israel. Strike where least expected. Do it when your adversary is confused or off balance. Feint him into a trap and then strike.

Yelling, shouting, screaming, howling a battle cry—all tend to unsettle an opponent and are time-honored ways of seizing the initiative in armed combat. Do not hesitate to do so when making an attack, especially an attack at close-quarters.

Diversion is another tactic that is used on the battlefield by generals or in a dark alley by someone who is suddenly attacked. Tossing a fistful of pennies, rocks, sand, etc., into your attacker's face will help you turn the tide of battle and maybe allow you to go on the attack yourself. Surprise is a time-honored tool of battle. Use it.

The Femoral Artery
This artery is under the groin. It is not a usual target, but it makes an excellent surprise target of opportunity. You can engage it by feinting a high attack, then bending low and slashing to the inside of your opponent's thigh. If you are

lucky, you will sever the artery and he will die within minutes. If you miss, you can still damage the inner thigh muscles severely and cripple your adversary.

The Auxiliary Artery
The auxiliary artery is located under the armpit, and if it is severed, death will occur in about 25 seconds. You can expose this vital area by circling your adversary, then suddenly reversing direction. This maneuver will almost always cause your enemy to raise his arm. Use the opportunity to slash him in the armpit.

The Kidney
You can hit the kidney by making your opponent attack you, then bending low and slipping by him, stabbing him in the side, then slicing your blade toward his kidney. This is followed by moving clear of him, circling, and watching as your enemy dies in about 25 seconds.

The Elbow
The elbow lends itself very well to filling the role of surprise target of opportunity. You should attack it when your enemy momentarily becomes careless. Slashing the elbow area almost anywhere will result in paralysis of the arm. You may get lucky and sever the ulnary artery, which will result in your enemy's death in a minute or two.

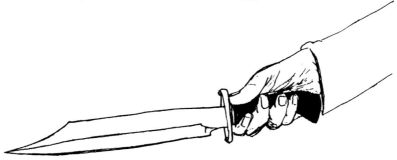

COMBAT KNIFE GRIP.

THE COMBAT KNIFE GRIP

There are many ways to hold a knife while eating. Europeans hold it in the weak hand and use it to press things like peas onto forks, never letting it out of their grasp. North Americans hold the knife in their strong hand and put it down after each use. But for deadly combat, there is only one way.

The combat knife grip gives you full control of the knife, yet allows you to handle it in an almost dancelike manner. You can slash, stab, chop with it, and never lose control or be forced to change your hand position on the knife. You can swing into a fast-forward slash, then move back into a backward slash without rotating your wrist if armed with a bowie with sharpened false edge or a double-edged fighting knife. You can deliver a blow with maximum leverage and power if you do not violate the principles of the time-proven combat knife grip.

Assuming the Combat Knife Grip

Place the knife handle diagonally across the palm of the strong hand, hilt parallel to the index finger, blade parallel to the thumb. Curl your fingers around the handle, then place your thumb along the handle top. Press the thumb forward up against the back of the hilt, and hold the handle in a firm, natural manner.

THE BASIC COMBAT KNIFE STANCE

"Float like a butterfly, sting like a bee." These famous lines sum up the key to the combat stance in a knife fight. To win, one has to be fast and agile, possessing the ability to deceive the opponent with a series of smooth reflex actions.

The correct combat stance in the circle of death must be suited for both defense and offense, because all knife combat is very much like a dance between these two very different tactics.

The torso must be held erect, balanced on slightly bent knees so that you are in a semicrouch, your head in a straight

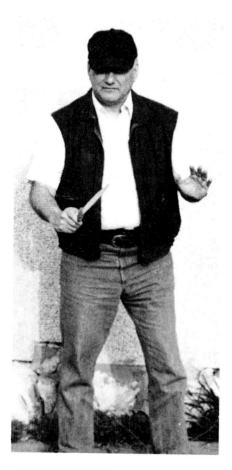

COMBAT KNIFE STANCE.

line with your chest. Your legs are comfortably spread so that the weight of the body is evenly distributed on them. If you are right-handed, then your left foot will be positioned slightly in front of the body. Hold the right hand partially forward, keeping the forearm slightly below chest level, parallel with the ground.

The knife arm elbow should be sort of cocked and in line with your chest, a few inches from your side. Keep your left hand extended forward, holding it at chest level so that it can fend off attack, or even grasp your opponent. You must never block a knife attack with your hand unless you absolutely have no choice.

If forced to ward off your opponent's knife, do it with the palm, an area of your hand that is much less likely to be crippled if you are cut. The old street tactic of wrapping your jacket around your weak hand and arm isn't a bad idea, since it will absorb some of your opponent's attack. A cut jacket is certainly better than cut tendons. Keep circling to your left, since this lets your left hand act as a shield while your right hand is ready to attack or counterattack. The left-sided circling motion keeps your left foot forward of the right and gives you an excellent platform for stepping forward with the left leg when launching an attack. It your attack is foiled, you can swiftly move back into a defensive position from which the attack can be resumed easily. The goal is to have superb balance while retaining the ability for swift, agile movement.

In order to confuse your opponent and keep him off balance, try to stay away from forming a tell-tale pattern in any fight, and certainly a knife fight. Stay loose; move like a butterfly. Keep your pattern of movement unpredictable. Circle, then shift the circle in another direction. Dart in and out, feinting all the time so as to fake your enemy into an unbalanced position from which he cannot defend himself if you decide to shift gears and attack suddenly. As when dancing, you must keep leading or you will find yourself being led.

When in the counterattack, remember that while the thrust can be used, it necessitates getting into your enemy's strike zone, where he then can counterattack. The problem with the thrust is that it must be delivered with sufficient force to be really effective. This means modifying your stance in one of two ways: you charge close enough to plunge your blade in, or you extend your knife arm and place your body weight behind the thrust. Charging close puts you in jeopardy. Extending your arm makes you lose balance and helps your enemy if he counterattacks.

Ideally, if you can sucker your enemy into doing just this, you can slice him to smithereens. Better use the extended arm thrust for faking your opponent out. The one exception is going for your opponent's throat, where a swift attack could put him out of the game. But this must be done quickly and be followed up with your withdrawal. When in the combat stance, remember that balance is the key to survival. Never use tactics that defeat this basic principle.

ATTACK!

We have spoken of attack. Now let us delve into the basis of this concept of street survival. Attack is the name of the game in combat, and never more than when in the circle of death. The man who attacks first in an aggressive and swift manner controls the fight. The erratic moving target of the attacker is certainly the most difficult target to engage. The initiative falls to the attacker who circles, reverses, feints, attacks, retreats, in a seemingly haphazard pattern that is controlled and flows with the battle. Attacking doesn't just mean blindly charging forward; it does mean controlling the battlefield in a fluid series of movements. It is not static. In knife fighting it means slashing your enemy to ribbons in a series of cuts aimed at the face, throat, chest, arms, stomach, and legs, choosing the vital targets in these areas if possible and the lesser targets if easier. Use retreat only as a prelude to an aggressive counterattack. Make your opponent fearful. Make him bleed. Make him immobile, then finish him off. In battle and out in the street, the best defense is an aggresive offense.

COUNTERATTACK!

You have been forced by circumstances to retreat temporarily to avoid your enemy's knife. You are alert to see if his attack has slowed down or if he blunders in some way, thus exposing himself to counterattack. To do this, you must be well trained, cool-headed, and have the intestinal fortitude to shift gears at the most opportune moment. Maybe it's a good time to use psychological warfare and fake fear and confusion . . . maybe even stupidity. The Plains Indians of the Wild West, Genghis Khan and his Golden Horde, all used fake retreat as a means of suckering their enemies into a false sense of confidence that the battle was almost over, thus making their enemies move at them with contempt, flush with victory, lowering their defenses. Suddenly, turning the tables, they would defeat their enemies in a vicious counterattack.

Retreating, the giving up of territory, makes sense when you maintain your balance and movement and are ready to counterattack swiftly at the moment you see an opening. Counterattack is really just attack in another form.

THE KING OF BLADED WEAPONS: THE SWORD

If I had to pick the most underappreciated yet formidable

weapon in existence today, it would be the sword. This is a sleeper in bladed weapons which must again take its place as king of the mountain. It is an ideal and quite legal weapon for home use in most locales. Swords have the advantage of being long, well-balanced, and, when razor-sharp, able to deliver slashing, chopping, and stabbing blows with equal ease and at a comfortable distance from one's adversary. Unfortunately, swords have all but been forgotten in our modern world. This shouldn't be the case. If I were not allowed to have a firearm in my home, the next weapon I would choose would be the sword.

While the short sword with blade of approximatly 19 inches will do, the broadsword is more to my liking. A blade of 31 to 37 inches helps "keep the wolf at bay."

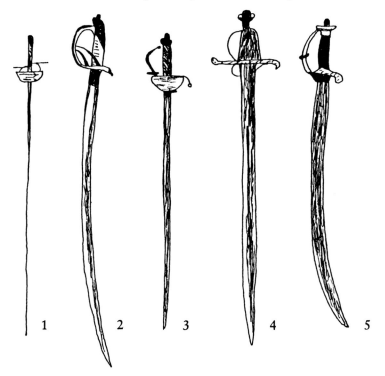

KING OF BLADED WEAPONS: 1. fencing foil, 2. saber, 3. rapier, 4. broadsword, 5. cutlass.

The cutlass with a blade of about 28 inches is also a good choice. The same with sabres of the 36-inch length. I don't like rapiers as much because their blades are a little on the thin side, though their length of 32 to 45 inches is quite adequate. Stay away from dueling foils, since they really are only best for piercing.

Swordplay

In training for the use of the sword, keep in mind that just about all books dealing with the subject consider dueling and fencing to be the only correct ways to use a sword. They only envision the conceptual use of sword against sword, duelist against duelist. None envision the use of the sword against a modern-day criminal predator armed with, say, a switchblade knife.

In viewing the sword for present-day use, one has to break long-held tradition and mind-set and reconsider it as a very long and well-balanced bowie knife. This is a mind-boggling jump for most people, though the concept is not so far-fetched as it first seems, since many historians consider the bowie knife as no more than a reduced-in-size and recontoured Roman short sword. Consider that the Roman short sword was the weapon that conquered the world, and you can see why the sword—any sword—is the most formidable bladed weapon ever devised.

In purchasing a sword, make sure you find one that is of good basic quality—no mean task. We are not speaking of poor-quality cane swords, some of which are really only long ice picks, but of large-bladed swords that are able to have their cutting edges honed to a razor sharpness, swords made of high-quality steel that won't break like glass rods when meeting the very firm resistance offered by heavy bone and muscle.

Since, for our purposes, we view the sword in a very different way from the conventional wisdom, considering it a very oversized bowie knife, the principles of knife fighting that we have discussed in the circle of death apply. For instance, you never want to strike from a position that raises the sword over your head, thus needlessly exposing your own anatomy to

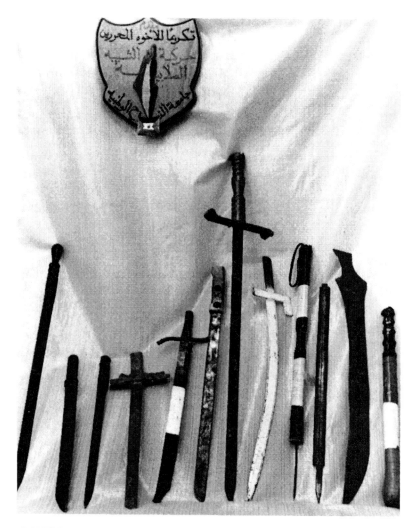

CAPTURED SWORDS OF THE PLO AND HAMAS: Such weapons, many homemade, are the favorite tools of assassins who murder fellow Arabs suspected of working for Israel.

swift counterattack. Rather, you want to slowly slice, chop (swords are excellent for this chore), and puncture your opponent into bloody submission in a very surgical and cold-blooded manner. Never rush at and into an opponent's defensive reach with your sword in hand. You don't have to. Getting close to an opponent puts you at a very needless and serious disadvantage. The sword gives you reach. Why squander that advantage foolishly? Against a correctly wielded sword, your adversary will experience a very unpleasant surprise if he attempts to grab its razor-sharp edge.

You have won invulnerable and valuable reach with the sword. The so-called long knife can make you a certain winner in any close-quarter fight as long as you are not up against a firearm.

The Sword Thrust

With the knife, even the bowie knife, the horizontal stabbing thrust is considered a very dangerous manuever since you enter your opponent's strike zone. This is not true with the sword because of its long blade length. The sword gives you reach without moving you into the highly dangerous area of your adversary's knife. This can make you a winner even against the most skilled street fighter armed with a knife.

The Sword Combat Stance

The use of the combat stance of the knife fighter will probably offend those who are skilled with the épée or foil and who duel in the highly stylized techniques of centuries past. New ideas and thinking always come up against previously accepted concepts. The idea of the sword being what the American Plains Indians called a long knife is such a new idea. Trained duelists should not see this as an attack on proven doctrine but rather as a very tailored new use of the sword for modern street survival.

Classical fencers and duelists are trained to present as little of their body to an opponent as possible when engaging in a duel with sword pitched against sword, turning sideways to avoid the thrusts of their opponent. This is now obsolete for the problems we envision with the sword. What we desire is flexibility of movement, since we have a monopoly on reach. The knife fighter's combat stance for the circle of death is the ideal.

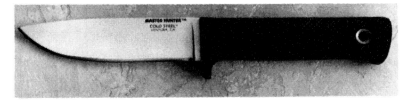

COLD STEEL MASTER HUNTER: While such knives can kill, their thick, broad, flat-ground 4 1/2-inch blades are better suited to field kitchen duties.

STREET SURVIVAL LESSONS

1) *Ambush with bladed weapons.* For ambushing, almost any type of bladed weapon will suffice.

2) *Classical knife fight.* In the circle of death, a 9- to 10-inch bowie knife is the ideal choice.

3) *Think attack and counterattack.* Know attack and counterattack techniques. Never let the enemy call how you respond to his attack.

4) *Be leery of your enemy at all times.* Always fight with a worst-case-scenario mentality. Never underestimate the capabilities of your enemy. Remember, he can also fake weakness, fear, and hesitation in combat as a ploy to sucker you.

5) *Beware your enemy's strike zone.* Never enter the strike zone of your opponent unless you are on the attack.

6) *Know when to break off an attack.* When on the attack, upon seeing that you are not succeeding, pull back. Assume the combat stance and prepare to counterattack at the first opportune moment.

7) *Draw blood.* Never have your enemy enter your strike zone without making him pay. Make him bleed, punish him, win a psychological point by making him fearful.

8) *Don't throw your weapon away.* Don't throw your knife at your enemy; you may arm him.

9) *Don't get fancy.* Don't toss your knife from hand to hand; you may drop it. And if you don't drop it, remember that a knife blow delivered with your weaker hand may not do severe damage.

10) *Float like a butterfly.* Keep your balance. Never lunge. Move one step at a time. Circle your enemy, evade, force the fight in the direction you deem fit.

11) *Sting like a bee.* An aggressive, sustained attack is the best defense. Strike fast and first. Carry the fight to your enemy. Seize and hold the initiative so that your opponent can't launch an attack.

12) *Controlled retreat.* If forced to retreat, do it in a controlled manner, waiting for the opportunity of counterattack to retake the initiative.

Case Study: Jerusalem Knife Attack

An Arab terrorist stabs a woman to death and runs down a street in Jerusalem. An Israeli police officer shouts for him to halt. The terrorist does not halt. Following police orders, the officer does not shoot to kill, but rather aims for the terrorist's legs with his NF Hi-Power pistol loaded with military ball ammo. The terrorist is hit and falls to the sidewalk. The officer does not then fire bullets into the terrorist's head but goes to him, and is attacked by the perp who, stabbing upward, plunges a butcher knife into him. The officer dies. The terrorist is apprehended by other officers who arrive on the scene.

This sad case, which occurred in the last year, is a classic learning exercise in how to get police officers needlessly killed. The problem was not in the officer's weapon, nor even in the choice of bullet. The problem was in the mental attitude of the police authorities who ordered the capture of terrorists.

STREET SURVIVAL LESSONS

1) *A live enemy is a dangerous enemy.* Even if you have severely wounded an assailant, remember he is still dangerous. Never move close, even if he is down. Don't grasp defeat out of the jaws of victory by letting your opponent kill you at the last moment. As long as your enemy breathes, he should be considered dangerous. Remember, he may be playing possum.

2) *Don't capture mad dogs.* Disabling shots are nonsense when firing at armed terrorists, psychopaths, and spaced-out drug addicts. Killing shots should have been fired.

3) *The weapon you don't see can kill you.* Obviously, the officer did not see the knife, or did he believe the terrorist was incapable of still attacking him?

Deadly Cold Weapons

In this chapter on cold weapons, I have attempted to sensitize the reader to the almost endless list of items that can be utilized by friend and foe alike. Throughout history, so-called cold weapons have probably resulted in the loss of more human life than even the much more efficient hot weapons of our modern age. Forewarned is forearmed. Even that innocuous garden rake can remove someone's eye or worse. The ingenuity of man is without bounds, the list of adhoc weapons he can employ seemingly endless.

Chapter Four

Street Weapons— "Hot"

*B*e not afraid of any man no matter
what his size. When danger threatens
call on me, and I will equalize.

—Author unknown

I once saw this famous poem carved
into an ivory grip of a heavily factory
engraved, silvered Colt single action .45
LC 5 1/2-inch-barreled pistol. If memory
serves me well, the gun was turned out in
the late 1800s. It was a masterpiece, and
though the poem has appeared in other
places, that particular gem of a firearm
still sticks in my mind. Owned by
Connecticut collector of fine firearms
Jonathan Peck, it was a deadly tool that
was transformed into a work of art with a
philosophy to live by carved into its grips.

I must admit to being extremely prej-
udiced when it comes to the use of
firearms for legitimate self-defense. No
invention has so revolutionized combat
as has gunpowder. For the first time in
history, the meek could inherit and protect the earth from predatory evil. While
it is true that the bow and crossbow
moved the common man in that direction, gunpowder completed the journey.

Today, it is inexcusable for anyone to be at the mercy of the strong and evil. That is what makes the antigun hysteria sweeping the United States so despicable. Denying the weak the best and sometimes only means to counter criminally superior force places the antigun lobby square in the camp of those who harm the weak and innocent. The antigun lobby becomes the unsuspecting ally of crime in the streets and so encourages its growth.

THE PRINCIPLE OF UNIFORMITY

As someone who has worked with thousands of soldiers, I venture to say I am the only man on earth who was given a paratroop brigade to train single-handedly. I have come to the firm conclusion that a rule I live by called the principle of uniformity is valid and critical for survival in conflict. I am convinced it can only help you under the stress of conflict; it certainly cannot get you killed.

The principle of uniformity is actually only a practical off-shoot of the time-honored concept that "what you train is what you do under stress." Mortal combat on the battlefield or in the street is simply controlled chaos in that whatever you have planned probably will go haywire when the moment of truth arrives. In all armed encounters, Murphy's Law is very much alive and kicking.

Under stress, we tend to do what we have been trained to do. I never could understand seemingly level-headed experts in the field of weaponry and tactics advising people on how they themselves carry a "snubby .38 Special in a rear pocket holster when off-duty and a .357 Magnum in a border patrol holster on the right hip when on duty." In one article, I read, "When I visited that foreign country, I carried a 9mmP Browning Hi-Power in a front cross-draw holster and a .380 in an ankle holster." In another, I read, "My Star PD feels right at home in my small-of-the-back holster along with the derringer I hid away in my hat."

Great balls of fire! You're a better man than me, Gunga Din. I'd be utterly confused. Imagine having to draw a primary and then a secondary weapon under stress while walking around in such a haphazard manner of carry. All this while a spaced-out drug addict in some dark parking lot or some "Khomeini Moro" wielding a blood-red ax charges at me? I get shivers up my spine just thinking about it.

Don't make life more complicated than it is. Keep it simple. Use the principle of uniformity to your advantage. Always carry your weapons, ammo, and equipment in the same body area. This is just as critical as the type of weapon you choose. Confusion under stress is a highly dangerous condition. Avoid it at all costs.

The type of holster you wear is not as critical as where you place it. For instance, whether you use a front cross-draw holster, a bellyband, a shoulder holster, or even a fanny pack, your hand will quickly compensate for the method of carry as long as the chosen carrying system is always kept in the same area of the body, namely, the front of your waist, the left side, or the right side. Once again, what you don't want to do is change the carrying position so that the holster is not where you would always expect it to be when you reach for your weapon. Keep whatever handgun, magazine, speed loader, or knife you'll want there all the time, and don't shift places. If you do, then the danger increases that under stress you may reach for a nonexistent item. For example, the use of an ankle holster is fine if you wear one all the time; not so if it is an occasional carry position. Don't play musical chairs with your life-support systems or you may find yourself a loser in the game called street survival.

Case Study: Jonathan on the Road

E.S.: Jon, I've explained the principle of uniformity to you. What is your assessment of the idea based on your years as a street cop, SWAT team member, and Ranger who now resides in the Wild Mideast?

J: It's a valid concept that has to be pushed. I recently had it impressed on me only a few weeks ago when I was driving up a road in what could be called "less than friendly territory." I sometimes am forced to do a lot of traveling on isolated roads in what the media calls the "West Bank" and what you and I call Judea and Samaria, the Biblical names. It is an area riddled with Islamic and PLO terrorists. A lone driver in a car traveling up a side road makes a tempting target.

E.S.: What were you carrying at the time?

J: I had a Glock 21 loaded with .45-caliber Speer 200-grain bullets—the so-called "flying ashtray" bullet. My SWAT team friends back in the United States have always been pleased with its effect on targets. I was carrying it in a strong-side holster when I saw the road blocked up ahead in what looked like a one-car accident. Four Arabs in their twenties were vigorously trying to flag me down. Since the road was blocked by their car, I was forced to slow down and instinctively reached for my pistol. It wasn't there! I suddenly realized I had always carried it in a shoulder holster (left side or a left front cross draw) for years, and when it looked like it was going to hit the fan, I reached for my handgun as I had done in dozens of firefights over the years. It wasn't there. If they had opened up on me, I probably wouldn't be talking to you now. I'd be dead with a heck of a surprised look on my face.

E.S.: Had you been practicing the strong-side [FBI] draw for long?

J: I thought I had, but when the balloon went up I unconsciously fell back on what I had practiced much more, the front cross draw. I did it without thinking, instinctively, concentrating instead on the danger I faced up ahead.

E.S.: Why did you switch?

J: I now carry openly, as many do in Israel, and I found that the strong-side carry attracted less attention since it seems to be the way almost 100 percent of the population chooses to carry pistols. I have now decided to go back to what is obviously deeply imprinted in my subconscious mind, the front cross draw. The social acceptance problem I now deem much less important than the street survival lesson I have learned.

E.S.: What happened with the car accident?

J: I decided four against one wasn't a very good set of odds to play with. Since they had chosen an area of the road for their car breakdown (the car's hood was up) that was isolated and did not allow me to pass by them or even to turn around, I jumped out with my Glock in hand, took cover, and covered them.

E.S.: Were they armed?

J: I never did find out. They slammed down the hood and all four of them jumped into their car, gunned the engine, and raced away. It seems the "car breakdown" had somehow miraculously cured itself.

I now carry my Glock 21 in a front cross draw or a shoulder holster on the same side as I did in my SWAT team days. You can line me up as a firm believer in the principle of uniformity. There is something to it. It's definitely not bullshit or writer's hype.

THE HANDGUN

Probably the best personal weapon around today is the handgun, primarily because you'll have it with you when danger strikes. The sound idea that a man chooses a rifle or shotgun when he goes to war is true; however, out there in the street the handgun still reigns supreme.

The Semiauto

The semiauto handgun offers higher magazine capacity as well as speed of reloading over the revolver. It also offers something in the way of concealment and comfort of carry when we are speaking of the larger models versus the larger revolvers.

Because they are cycled by the gasses generated by the burning of gunpowder, they are more prone to easily cleared stoppages (not full-blown handgun jams) due to ammunition sensitivity.

Case Study: No Gun Stores in Sight

Baum tells an anecdote about his raid into Egypt that points out the need of checking your carry ammo (especially for semiauto handguns) whether for war or in the street.

E.S.: Before you went on that famous commando raid into Egypt, what precautions did you take?

B: Many, but one is pertinent to our learning street survival. Remember, we were entering enemy territory with a small armored commando force. For all intents and purposes, except for some air cover, we were on our own. We had to make do with what we had, much like someone walking in a deserted street at night. I had ordered tens of thousands of rounds of new .50-caliber ammo for our heavy machine guns. A few days before we embarked on the raid, the ammo arrived in factory-new boxes. I asked the men in charge of the shipment if they had checked it out. They assured me the factory standards were of the highest degree possible, and they had no worries about the quality of the ammo.

E.S.: Did you share their opinion?

B: They were correct, of course, if I was going on a training exercise in our southern desert, the Negev. However, I am a firm believer in worst-case-scenario planning, so I broke open some of the boxes and proceeded to fire-test the ammo.

E.S.: Were the ordnance people right?

B: Dead wrong. I had nothing but primers popping when I pulled the trigger on some of the rounds. I pulled the bullets to find empty cases. It seems for the first time ever the gunpowder did not drop into the cases and somehow got past inspection. For all intents and purposes, we had no ammo. We would have found that out in a firefight deep behind enemy lines. The factory boys were red-faced and tongue-tied, a condition I preferred to our being purple-faced dead, tongues blackening in the Egyptian sun. The double tragedy is probably no one would have known why the commando raid was a failure if we were all killed. *Always check your ammo as if your life depended on it.* It does.

....

STREET SURVIVAL LESSONS

1) *Believe no one when your life is at stake.* All equipment should be checked and then double-

checked on a routine basis. Semiauto guns and ammo are especially sensitive to problems.

2)   *Do it yourself.* All inspections should be carried out by you, even if the experts assure you everything is in perfect working order. Worst-case-scenario planning can save your life. A firefight is no place to find bugs in your equipment.

Conditions of Carry: 1, 2, 3, 4

I have almost always carried Colt 1911 autos or their clones as my street guns. This in the condition #1 cocked and locked mode. Nothing points and feels better in my hand than these Colts, unless it's a good Smith and Wesson or Ruger double-action revolver with proper grips. (Sorry, I just don't like the trigger action on Colt revolvers, not even a Python, and I've owned more than a few.)

One of the big mistakes for street carry is to carry a single-action semiauto in conditions #2, #3, and, of course, #4.

Condition #2, hammer down on a live chambered round, means you have to thumb-cock the hammer like a "cowboy pistol"—not a very clever idea when you realize that the hammer on most single-action semiautos is not really designed for that rather delicate task (not to mention that you have to lower it on a live round to put it into that position in the first place).

Condition #3 is very popular here in Israel and is, in my opinion, a dead-wrong system of carry. Having to rack a slide back to load a handgun necessitates two hands and turns your handgun into a "hands gun." Imagine trying to do this while warding off a knife-wielding enemy. The hair on the back of my neck stands up at the thought. I know for a fact that this ridiculous method of carry has resulted in the death of numerous Israelis, good men cut down by close-quarter attackers armed with axes and knives. That this impossible system works at all here in Israel is a tribute to the quality of the men and not to the carry method of condition #3.

For those of you who are skeptical about my opinion of condition #3, I offer you an exercise I developed called "Knock the Old Lady Down." I developed this exercise for a group of Israeli settlers living in the ancient city of Hebron, an area mentioned in the Bible as having been purchased by Abraham. These settlers walk through dark alleys and open food markets, rubbing shoulders with potential knife-, ax-, and, recently, gun-toting terrorists. In such a situation, quick response to attack is the key to street survival. One hand may be needed to ward off an attack, a much more important task than needlessly using said hand to rack back a slide. Because of this, I developed a simple, practical street survival exercise that brings cruel reality home to believers of condition #3.

Place a full-sized silhouette target in front of you at just about contact distance. Call this target the old lady. Now place a second target behind the old lady. Call this target a berserk knife-wielder. Face the old lady with your semiauto pistol holstered and in condition #3. To make things more interesting and realistic, hold a shopping bag in each hand filled with glass bottles and jars. After all, this is supposed to be an open-air market, isn't it?

Now have a friend shout, "Terrorist!" You let the bags drop from your hand, not an easy task when we consider the fact that since birth we have been ingrained with the statement "Don't drop that." Push the old lady aside with your weak hand while you draw your pistol with your strong hand. Engage the terrorist by firing a triple tap. All this must be done in under 1.5 seconds.

I had a security guy on my range who argued the merits of condition #3 carry. I told him not to argue but rather do the exercise any way he liked—cocked and locked or empty chamber. Needless to say, he now carries his pistol in condition #1, cocked and locked. He had his eyes opened. It was only an exercise, the best place to learn. Learning out in the street can be detrimental to one's health.

Condition #4 is carrying your pistol empty with the magazine out. This may make sense for storage of one's handgun at home. It makes no sense outside the home, for the obvious reason that it's much too slow and necessitates using two hands to load your pistol. I doubt that very many people carry their handguns that way, though one sees everything out in the street.

In my opinion, the single-action auto is the ideal street gun, since it is easy to carry, points well, shoots fast and accurate, and is quick to reload. Most competition pistols are of this design because of these qualities.

The Thumb Switch

The ambidextrous thumb safety is an excellent way to get the cocked and locked semiauto into fire-ready condition when a right-handed shooter is forced to draw the pistol with his left hand. Certainly, having the handgun ready for use with either hand is a basic need in street survival. Just ask Luke Short, a man who killed some of the toughest gunmen in the West but never did get the fame he deserved. The greatest shoot-out Short ever was in was against "Texas Jim Courtwright," a Lone Star state peace officer and gunman supreme. Courtwright was the ten-to-one favorite when the duel commenced—that is, until Short's first bullet nearly severed Courtwright's thumb from his right hand, making it impossible for him to thumb-cock his single-action peace-

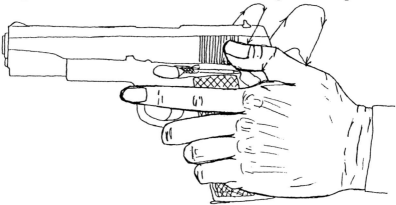

THUMB SWITCH: *The weak hand thumb is switched over the hammer to the hammer safety, the safety is pressed down, then the thumb is returned back over the hammer to the opposite side.*

maker. Before Texas Jim could do the border shift to his left hand (throwing the pistol to that hand), Short aimed and finished the great gunman off with the next bullet.

The story isn't exactly fitted to flipping off the hammer safety of a semiauto with the weak hand, but it does point out the direction of the dangers if one can't. What if one does not have an ambidextrous thumb safety? (You should.) Some say that a good technique is to flip off the safety with the weak hand's forefinger while the gun is still in the holster. I don't like that because if I'm in a fight for my life, I want to get that gun out fast, and flipping its safety off before I draw it is too slow. Better to draw the gun and, as I bring it to bear, do what I have named the "thumb switch," bringing the weak hand's thumb over the hammer to flip off the safety, all the time keeping a tight grip on the handgun. The thumb switch is a natural.

STREET SURVIVAL LESSONS

1) *Keep a handgun.* Use condition #1, not condition #3.

2) *Thumb switch.* The thumb switch technique is faster than the weak forefinger technique for getting the thumb safety off.

The Double-Action Semiauto

While lauded as a new thing by those who should know better, the design is an old one (like most of what passes for new these days), going back to the turn of the century.

I find the criticisms of the design fair and valid. The first double-action trigger squeeze followed by a second semiaction trigger squeeze is somewhat detrimental to smooth and consistent manipulation of the trigger, and accuracy must suffer. That is not to say that it suffers drastically, and many shooters find this criticism a bunch of bull, declaring that they can blow the center out of a target on demand and doing just that.

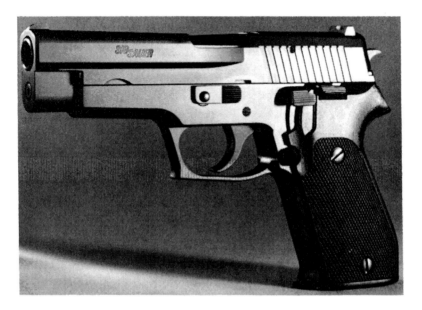

SIG SAUER P220 "AMERICAN" AUTO PISTOL: One of the better .45 ACP double-action autos.

If I had to carry such a pistol, I would sleep very well at night. It's just that in my hands I find the 100-percent single-action system more accurate. Since every little bit helps in close-quarter combat, why create needless obstacles between you and success? It's like carrying excessively hot ammo in the larger calibers. For an alleged increase in stopping power, one gets much more recoil and loss of smoothness in engaging multiple targets in a fast and furious shoot-out. After carrying such ammo and testing the effect on the range, I came to the conclusion it was more important to hit multiple targets with ease than get an alleged increase in actual stopping power. After all, fast and furious target impact is the basis of all gunfights. However, what works for one sometimes doesn't work for another. There are no absolutes in this business, and anyone who insists there are is tempting fate.

Glock has come out with a trigger system (also not new) that somewhat resembles a double-action revolver, giving the same "trigger feel" for each shot. We have also seen double-action-only (DOA) trigger systems that do the same thing, though usually with more force needed to work the trigger system. Once again, this is an art, not a science. Try them all. If one system works best for you, then by all means stick with it. But, remember, hits on target should be the ultimate measure of what works.

High Capacity?

I went to Colonel Baum on this one because he's probably been in more close-quarter gunfights than just about anyone alive today.

E.S.: What is your opinion of having a high capacity in a pistol? Say 14 to 20 rounds as compared to 6 to 9 rounds?

S.B.: It's not something that should be considered a frivolity, but rather a good combat principle. This is not to

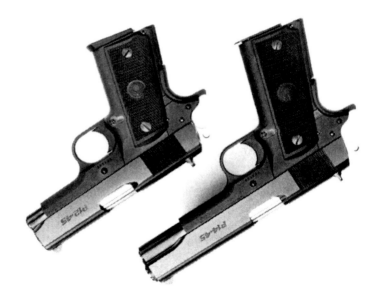

PARA-ORDNANCE P14-45 AND P12-45: High-capacity for those wanting more firepower in .45 ACP.

say that standard-capacity pistols are obsolete, far from that. Most pistol fights have been won with standard-capacity handguns. Tactics and cover plus good shot placement are still the most important things. That said, it's still nice to have a good supply of ammo in the handgun, or any gun for that matter. One less thing to bother with—that of changing your magazine in the heat of battle. I am for higher capacity in principle, though I wouldn't worry about it and have and do carry both types.

Let me ask you the same question, Gene. What do you find to be the best for you?

E.S.: Well, since I carry the .45 ACP semiauto in the street, I prefer the standard-capacity handgun in my hand, simply because it points better in point fire. This is especially true when I try firing a Glock 21 or the older-design Caspian Arms or Para-Ordnance handguns. They, especially the Glock, feel a little thick, and I find my index of deflection and "instinctive feel" are hampered a little by this. Of course, the situation could improve with use, and I am not giving you my final word on the matter. With new Para-Ordnance and Caspian Arms models, this is a moot point anyway, since they have recently placed standard grip, high-capacity models on the market. Now here is something that gives one the best of both worlds, high-capacity plus a very tried-and-true point-fire capability. Word is the trend in this direction is on the upswing, with more manufacturers jumping on the bandwagon.

High-Capacity

I like double-action revolvers. I like the fact that they fire any shape bullet with ease . . . that they can move a new cartridge into line if one misfires . . . that they point extremely well . . . that they are not dependent on their ammunition for reliability. What I don't like about them is that most carry only five or six rounds, and if they jam they are more difficult to get back into action than a self-loader. My wife Cynthia carries a S&W 1917 that I personally cut down for her, rounding off the grip and shortening the barrel to 3 inches. I then had it coated with BLACK-T, and she now carries it in a

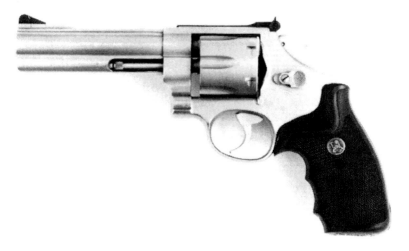

S&W MODEL 625-2: With full-moon clips, this revolver reloads at nearly auto magazine speed.

fanny pack. I can't seem to get her to carry a second revolver, but I have gotten her to carry three extra reloads. She shoots well. She never leaves our home without it since one of the women in our village was strangled (she survived) at the bus stop a few hundred yards down the road. Seems the attacker bungled the job.

You can get around some of the negative things about revolvers by carrying two of them out in the street and making them both .45 ACP (or 9mmP if you insist) so that they take the full-moon clip reloads. Other caliber options may be down the pike. These full-moon clips are the greatest thing going for revolvers since double action. Sure, speed loaders are good, but these full mooners are better, I think much better.

The Single-Action Revolver

The single-action revolver should really be regulated to sport use only, since it is just too slow to eject its empties and reload. I suppose a pair of them in the street could do the trick most of the time, but I think you are just being a glutton for punishment if you decide to carry them. Out in low-crime country (if such a place still exists) and on horseback, it does have its place in good hands. But those hands are far and few between. I do have a case of a single-action stopping a terrorist dead in his tracks. But remember, one swallow doesn't mean spring is around the corner.

Case Study: Single Action vs. Terrorists

A few years back up in the north of Israel, two terrorists landed by boat from the Mediterranean Sea. They came upon a father and his little daughter. As he pleaded for her, they bashed her brains out in front of his eyes, then shot him (he lived) and proceeded to a block of apartments. Entering it, they smashed in doors and entered one apartment, where a mother hiding in the closet with her infant inadvertently smothered it as she sat hidden in the darkness. Next, they pounded on the door of an apartment where a recent immigrant from the Republic of South Africa lived. He grabbed a Ruger Single-Six with his magnum cylinder in it and shot a terrorist through a very thin front door. The terrorist dropped dead. The Israeli antiterrorist unit arriving on the scene killed the other terrorist.

It seems the immigrant had no license for his handgun. Because of his heroic actions, no charges were filed and he was quietly given a gun license.

STREET SURVIVAL LESSONS

1) *Always be armed.* Hindsight shows that had the father had a firearm, things might have turned out differently. Even on that quiet beach, "sea monsters" came out of the ocean and went on a rampage of death.

2) *Any gun is better than no gun.* In a pinch, any design of gun is better than no gun at all. That little single-action Ruger saved many lives.

The Derringer

Since the assassination of President Abraham Lincoln, the derringer has enjoyed a quasimysterious status as a handgun. This, coupled with its depiction in Wild West films as a pistol that can decisively settle a fight across a card table, has given it a reputation as a fighting weapon that it does not rightly deserve.

Most derringers are two-barreled jobs, though single-shot models were also popular in this gun's heyday, and four-barreled models have also been seen. These add lots of bulk to a pistol supposedly chosen for lack of bulk. About the only strong suit of most derringers is their diminutive size. This attribute is far outweighed by their small cartridge capacity. Even if you choose a modern double-action model rather than the classical single-action design, the small capacity and slow reloading characteristics weigh against choosing it as a primary or secondary street weapon. While it could be used as a tertiary weapon, there are so many other superior designs of handguns around that it would seem to be a very poor choice.

Never base your choice of weaponry on nostalgia—this is a totally useless commodity in a firefight. Choices made on emotion rather than logic can get you killed. Personally, I'd pass on derringers for the street; they just don't fill the bill. Keep them for daydreaming, play, and nostalgia, not for the ordeal and nightmare of an armed confrontation.

Backup Handgun

The handgun's portability and easy concealment make it the everyday street weapon of choice, and what is said for one handgun goes double for two. Many old-time gunfighters carried a brace of matching pistols. I've always considered the idea as one having lots of merit, especially when the second handgun is of the same caliber as the first and the magazines or speed loaders are interchangeable.

Always try to have the principle of uniformity on your side, and this applies to handguns and ammunition. Why carry a .45 ACP as a primary weapon and then choose a .38

Special as a secondary weapon? If your primary weapon is lost in a shuffle out there in the street or, following Murphy's Law, its firing pin cracks on you, you would automatically make its ammunition quite useless, as your .38 snubby obviously could not digest the big .45 round you have in those extra magazines. Except for their dubious use as hand-thrown missiles, they would only be so many useless weights on your body.

A backup handgun is always there, providing a psychological boost in that, as with all backup systems, you don't feel totally dependent on the one and only system functioning reliably.

Ideally, the backup handgun should be instantly available to either hand, though circumstances and cultures in different locales may deem otherwise. The main problem is usually that of maintaining concealability. For example, here in Israel, it is quite acceptable to carry a handgun on the strong side. But if you carry it in a front cross draw, it elicits looks and such questions as, "What is this, Texas?" The same would be true if a second handgun were seen. However, believe it or not, if you strung an Uzi over your shoulder along with your handgun, no one would even notice.

Cultural acceptability can be a very real problem out in the street and may force us to sometimes make compromises we don't like, depending on and tailored to what country we live in.

Don't make light of the problem; it's very real. For instance, carrying a semiauto cocked and locked and in plain sight here in Israel is deemed dangerous by some and can actually get you into an argument or worse.

Recently, I broke both local taboos by carrying out a personal test of keeping my primary handgun cocked and locked in a front-cross-draw holster. My backup was hidden in a gunnysack strung onto my strong side. When my wife and I exited a "working man's" restaurant, an establishment known only for its excellent Mideast fast food cuisine and not for its decor, five local guys spotted my Colt sitting snug inside a front-cross holster. They had a quick conversation,

and one jumped up and challenged me with a most unfriendly, "Why are you carrying that pistol that way?" I informed
him it was quite safe, even going as far as to explain it all in
detail. He grew angrier and angrier and demanded I put it
into condition #3. I, of course, politely refused, which
enraged him even further. He shouted for some ID, wanting
to report me to the police. I got a little hot under the collar
and proceeded to question his parentage and knowledge of
firearms. That seemed to put a damper on his enthusiasm,
and I walked off, my enjoyment of an otherwise quite tasty
meal ruined. I deemed the test a success in that I learned
another lesson for the street.

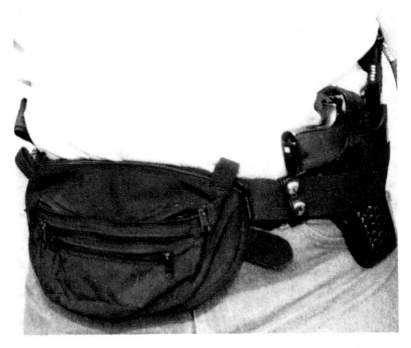

*.44 HOLSTER AND FANNY PACK. A .45 auto in condition #1 has its
hammer covered by the thumb snap on a .44 holster while another .45
sits hidden in a fanny pack. The rig takes into consideration the present
cultural norms of Israel and does not raise any eyebrows.*

Solving a Cultural Problem

The ways things are done vary with the area you live in. When you find that local conditions, no matter how ridiculous, interfere with your street survival options, it's time for some ingenuity and inventiveness. Answers can be found to almost all problems if you are willing to spend some time to think on and experiment with getting around them.

I wanted to carry my Colts in condition #1 and yet didn't want to alarm anyone who considered such a carry unsafe. I worked on the problem of open carry and came up with a workable solution: I found that if I carried my front-cross-draw pistol outside my shirt or jacket, I could still carry it cocked and locked in condition #1 if I ensconced it inside a quite different and unlikely holster, a Safariland #29 that is designed to carry a S&W .44 Magnum revolver with a 4-inch barrel.

With a reworked backstrap, the holster now tilts the 1911 or Commander into my hand. The Colts fit perfectly in it. The top retention snap doesn't close, but I don't care since I use it to cover the cocked and locked hammer with the holster outside the vest, jacket, or shirt. I have found this an ingenious solution to a very stupid but very real social problem. Meanwhile, I am working, writing, and lecturing, attempting to change negative attitudes against condition #1 carry in a country that needs the system more than most in the world.

STREET SURVIVAL LESSONS

1) *Don't draw attention to yourself.* Avoid going against local customs in dress and firearms display. "In Rome, do as the Romans do." Drawing needless attention to yourself may only excite the natives and cause rather than cure problems. Dress so as to blend in rather than stand out. Think of other ways to solve a cultural problem and still not compromise street survival principles.

2) *Use ingenuity.* When faced with a problem that
    you feel decreases your chances of street survival,
    remember the example I gave you, and see if you
    can't solve it by unorthodox methods. Never com-
    promise principles when survival is at stake.

3) *Familiarity breeds success.* Remember the principle
    of uniformity and do not vary the way you have
    your handgun ready for action (e.g., carrying a
    semiauto in condition #1 when concealed and in
    condition #3 when carrying openly). Varying the
    way your handgun is readied for action is just as
    dangerous as varying the place in which you keep it.
    Drawing an unloaded handgun can get you killed.

Noncompatible Handgun as a Backup

If finances or local laws mean you must carry a noncom-
patible handgun for a backup, you are almost always better
off in choosing a totally different system than that of the primary handgun. At first thought, this may seem nonsensical,
but I can assure you it is not. Like most things in life, there
are correct ways to do things and incorrect ways. Knowing
the difference can mean life or death. Such detailed thinking
is what separates the pro from the rank amateur.

For example, let us say you have chosen a Colt .45 auto as
your primary handgun and a 9mmP Beretta Model 92 as
backup. In making this choice, you have mixed a single-action
system with a double-action system—not a very big problem,
though it can lead to confusion under stress. We have already
addressed the problem of ammunition incompatibility. If your
Colt is put out of commission, then all the ammo for it is rendered as useless as marbles in your pocket. All of this you may
be able to live with, but you may not survive the problem of
attempting to insert a Colt magazine into your Beretta. The
problem with this mistake, especially at night, is that it may
take you too long to figure out what has happened. Such an
error could cost you your life out there in the street.

Locking Magazine Mix-Up

There is even a more dangerous scenario that can occur, that of using pistols of the same manufacturer that really accept magazines of different calibers, e.g., inserting and locking a Colt 9mmP magazine into a Colt .45 auto. I promise you, do such a thing and you may never know what went wrong before it's all over. Seeing the magazine insert and then lock will clear the brain of any worry that the wrong magazine has been inserted. Though I mentioned Colt as an example, there are other brands that I venture to say will do the same.

Make the Contrast Vivid

If you must carry an incompatible handgun as a backup, you are always better off choosing a totally different system, such as a revolver instead of another semiauto. This helps to eliminate deadly mix-ups. Of course, still strive for matching ammo.

If all this is not feasible and you have two closely related systems (two revolvers or two semiautos), remember to carry both sets of ammunition and carriers as far away from each other as possible. For example, carry your .45 ammo on your belt and your .9mmP ammo in a special pouch system on your ankle or in a gunnysack. Do this in a uniform manner. Don't vary anything. To do otherwise is tempting fate. Keep life simple. It's too complicated as it is. Always eliminate as many worst-case-scenario problems as you can before they occur.

....

STREET SURVIVAL LESSONS

1) *A brace of matching handguns.* Have your backup handgun be an exact duplicate of your primary one.

2) *Nonmatching backup.* If your backup can't match your primary handgun, have it be an exact opposite (revolver vs. semiauto). Even in this case, strive for ammo uniformity.

3) *Both handguns of same design.* When your back-up is of the same basic design as your primary handgun (two nonmatching revolvers or autos), keep the two types of ammo far apart.

....

The Third Handgun

For those in need of a third handgun (tertiary weapon), the principle of uniformity can be watered down. Why? Because a third handgun is usually one that places easy portability and concealment (a hideout) or specialty use (a handgun that accomplishes a special task) ahead of anything else. Caliber, number of rounds, and interchangeability of magazine or speed loaders are not as critical. But again, this is true only for a third handgun, not for the brace of handguns that form the basis of the fire system you carry out there in harm's way. Having your third handgun caliber and design compatible with your primary and backup guns is probably gilding the lily, though if it can be done, why not? But it should never be done at the expense of concealment and portability, which are the principle needs of the man carrying a third handgun.

Carrying a third handgun may not be as ridiculous as some may believe. A third pistol that is small can act as a hide-away—so-called onion field insurance. Or, it can be a standard size handgun that can do other tasks, such as filling the role of a long gun that is unavailable—sort of a mini carbine for long-distance shooting. Or, say it's a handgun that can handle special-purpose ammo for special tasks. The list is endless.

What applies to the third handgun applies to any fourth handgun carried. I have carried such a number of handguns myself on special occasions (circumstances deemed long gun carry inappropriate) and know others who have done the same.

Ideally, under the rule of uniformity, the third handgun should be of the same type and caliber as the primary and secondary ones. But this is not critical, since it is a third handgun and we can live with a little bending of the rules. This applies to any fourth handgun as well.

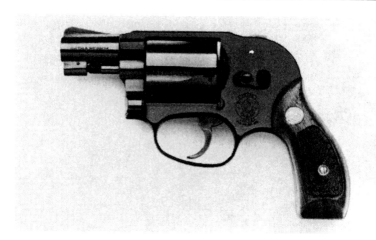

S&W MODEL 38 BODYGUARD: A 2-inch-barreled snubby that makes an excellent .38 Special pocket gun.

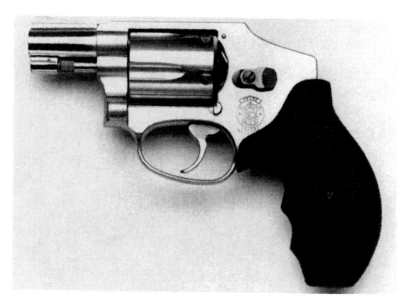

S&W CENTENNIAL 9MMP: A 2-inch-barreled snubby that uses the ballistically efficient 9mmP cartridge. Using full moon clips, it is considered by some to be the best medium-caliber pocket gun made.

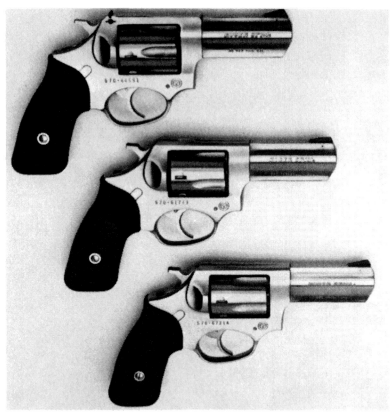

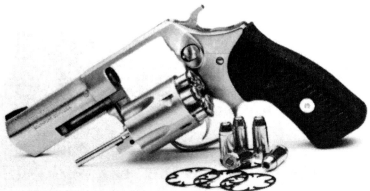

RUGER SP101: This powerfully built handgun is built to take .357 Magnum loads. It also uses the 9mmP in full moon clips.

On occasion. my choice of a third handgun has been a S&W .38-caliber snubby (I prefer the lightweight Bodyguard), since it delivers a very convincing projectile. I wish Smith & Wesson would come out with a larger five-shot version in .45 ACP that loads with five-cartridge full-moon clips. There is a need for such a handgun.

I have carried even the lowly .25 ACP handgun on occasion (settling it in as a fourth handgun). A friend presented me with a CZ model that is double-action and holds nine rounds. If forced into a wrestling match with an enemy out in the street—a match that placed my adversary's anatomy, and particularly his head, within powder burn distance—I do know how to eliminate such a threat. Of course, with the .25 I would assume I had a need to draw the weapon, since my hands should hopefully be able to draw my more deadly handguns. However, with worst-case-scenario planning that focuses on the remote possibility of such occurrences or even the unlikely event of my capture, the .25 may have a use. For this, one needs a good working knowledge of human anatomy. Such knowledge is critical if victory, and not defeat, is to be wrested from impending doom.

At contact distance, even the lowly and maligned .25-caliber will do the job if you know where to place its tiny projectile. Ask any farmer or slaughterhouse worker how a .22 short can bring down a steer with one well-placed shot to the brain and you will be convinced that it can be done even by the so-called mouse guns.

ANATOMICAL WEAK POINTS
OF THE HUMAN SKULL

Since the human brain is a very available target when you are rolling on the ground or standing and wrestling with your attacker, it becomes a prime target for your handgun, especially if said handgun is of diminutive caliber. Since the human brain is encapsulated in very heavy bone that acts as a sort of helmet, protecting it from lethal missiles, we must know the weak points of this defense system

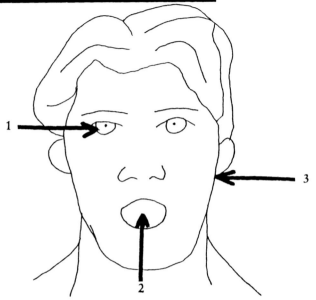

MOUSE GUN HEAD TARGETS—FRONTAL VIEW:
1. eye, 2. open mouth, 3. back of the ear.

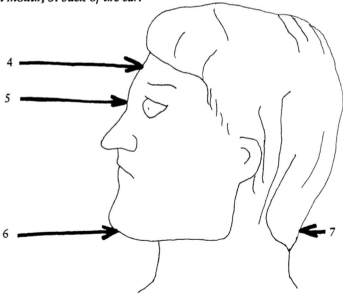

MOUSE GUN HEAD TARGETS—SIDE VIEW: 4. forehead, 5. between
the eyes, 6. base of chin, 7. medulla oblongata.

so as to be able to breach it. The area where the T of the T-ZONE is crossed is our target.

Ultimate Head Target: The Medulla Oblongata

At the rear of the neck, the spinal cord widens and moves into the base of the brain. This area of heavy cordlike nervous tissue is called the medulla oblongata. It is a prime target because cutting it turns off the electrical power from the brain to the body and results in instant shutdown without the danger of your enemy's trigger finger twitching in death and firing his weapon. The only handgun caliber that may not always penetrate deep enough to cut the medulla oblongata is the .25 (6.35mm) auto (if loaded with conventional 50-grain jacketed bullets at 810 fps). For this caliber, we can utilize only two pathways with some degree of certainty: a straight shot directed into the rear of the head where the spine joins the skull and under the front of the chin at a slight upward angle directed toward the spine.

A straight shot directed into the rear of the skull in the area where the spinal cord connects to the brain (the area of the medulla oblongata) is almost certain to do the trick. Firing directly into the medulla oblongata itself eliminates the need to penetrate heavy muscle or bone.

Frontally directing the muzzle of your pistol under your opponent's chin and at a slight upward angle should propel even the .25 projectile up into the spine for quick results.

The Open Mouth

A good route that can be utilized in breaching the body's defense system is the center shot through your enemy's open mouth. While such an opportunity is not too likely, you should be aware to capitalize on it if it exists. Such a shot, favored by many suicides, will send the handgun projectile directly into the brain (the .25 doesn't like this route; there is usually too much flesh and bone there for it to reach the brain).

Square Between the Eyes

A shot directed between the eyes has always been the ultimate target for fictional writers of action and crime films, and they are right. A bullet that hits this area will track directly into the brain and result in instant shut-down of the central nervous system. For best results, fire at a slight downward angle, avoiding the heavy bony ridge above the eyes (another route to avoid if your handgun is a .25).

The Ear

This also has been a target favored by film makers, and a correct one at that. How many times have we seen an officer in charge of a firing squad administer the coup de grace with a shot behind a prisoner's ear? For best results, the bullet should be placed about an inch down from the ear canal and a half inch toward the rear of the skull. Anything approximating this should do very nicely with all handgun calibers except the .25, which may or may not prove disappointing.

The Temple

The side of the forehead is an area where the bone is slightly thinner and so is a good area to direct your shot. Sorry, once again, this one is not recommended for the .25.

The Eye Socket

This is another area of the human skull that allows easier bone penetration and subsequent violation of the brain. Again, the .25-caliber may not perform satisfactorily.

NOTE: Both the temple and eye socket shot can kill your enemy, but it must be noted that these areas have one drawback. They may cause a reflex action that results in the trigger finger twitching in death and firing a firearm your enemy may have clutched in his hand.

The Ultimate Target

Even when using much more powerful weapons, Israeli police and military counterterrorist (CT) units have always considered the human head (and neck) a top-priority target. At 100 yards or less, it is the target of choice for snipers. However, except at almost contact distance, it may prove difficult to hit with a handgun. After all, your enemy won't be standing there like a static paper target on the range. The target may be moving and firing a weapon. Because of this, beyond almost-contact distance they aim for the center of mass. Hits count, not misses. However, once at contact distance, Israeli SWAT teams, never satisfied with halfway measures, repeatedly shoot the target's head until it is perforated like a sieve. They fire until their adversary is finished and can do no further harm. We would do well to remember these principles.

STREET SURVIVAL LESSONS

1) *The third (and fourth) handgun.* Circumstances may dictate the use of a third, or even fourth, handgun.

2) *Know your human anatomy.* Small calibers can prove very effective for close-quarter brain shots when one has a good working knowledge of the weak points in the human skull.

3) *Know your "mouse gun."* Know the limitations of your pistol when it is a .25 ACP (and most likely any of the .22-calibers that are standard velocity and fired from short barrels).

4) *Pump bullets.* Do as the Israeli elite units do when engaging a single target—pump the target with as many bullets as you can until your adversary is down and out of action. This includes contact-distance head shots.

WINNING THE CLOSE-QUARTER ENCOUNTER

Statistics have proven conclusively that the vast majority of street altercations take place from contact distance to 8 yards, with 1 yard being most common. Since a knife-wielding attacker can close the distance of 8 yards in less than 1.5 seconds, faster than most men can draw their handgun, the problem of street survival becomes acute.

In face-to-face encounters of the lethal kind, your first reaction should be to distract your opponent so that you can get your weapon into play before you are crippled or worse. Your weak hand is the key to this exercise and must be used for forcibly pushing and warding off your attacker. You push because you want to widen the distance again between you and your attacker. Here is where martial arts training will hold you in good stead as a prelude to your use of a handgun.

Logic and all the experts agree that a weapon in hand is the only way one can cut down the chances of getting cut. I have advised my students to do just that when they walk in areas infested with potential terrorists. I have kept the handgun under a vest, "Napoleon style," ready for instant use.

Case Study: Gun in Hand Worth Two Holsters

There is a famous cave called Machpela, which is covered by a huge building where Abraham and his family are buried. Going there one day proved to me the soundness of the gun-in-the-hand carry. When we left the building, my wife and I walked toward a bus stop that was quite far from where Israeli soldiers stood guard.

On the way to the bus, we suddenly felt alone and isolated as I noticed three young toughs making for us in a most suspicious manner. The area is known for being one where murderous attacks occur. I stopped, pulled my wife behind me, and, using body language (my hand under my jacket) and strong eye contact, sent out a clear message. Amazing how these things sometimes work like a charm.

The Arabs glared at my hand under my jacket, stopped dead in their tracks, and, reversing direction, walked off mumbling, all the time giving me most unfriendly looks.

Along with martial arts and weaponry, do not forget body language and correct mind-set. A strong subliminal message will many times be picked up. Most bullies are cowards, picking their victims from among the weak and unwary, just as predators in nature. When they smell trouble, they sometimes back off, seeking easier victims.

However, when they don't accommodate you and continue closing the distance between you and them, you must prepare to get your weapon into play. You have to go on the offensive. Never believe the ability to quick-draw your weapon in itself will be enough to settle any altercation. A close-range determined attack, especially by young men who are in excellent physical condition and under the influence of drugs or religious fanaticism, can be an awesome thing to encounter. Only an explosive counterattack coupled with controlled anger and accompanied by surprise can turn the tide of battle in your favor. Surprise, coupled with bold action, wins.

At the bus stop we were engulfed by literally hundreds of Arabs coming from school and places of work. We were there with four other Israelis—three elderly women and a man—all unarmed. One elderly lady looked around and asked, "I suppose no one has a gun around here do they?" I pulled back the vest slightly and she smiled (talk about a calming effect).

....

STREET SURVIVAL LESSONS

1) *Gun in hand wins.* When walking in elbow-rubbing distance of potential killers, nothing is better than a handgun in hand, ready for instant use.

2) *Use body language and eye contact to deter aggression.* If you feel an attack is possible, the use of body language and eye contact may discourage a predator bent on easy pickings.

....

Two Blocking Motions
One of the best blocking motions to ward off a point-range attacker is the circular sweep. This is executed with the

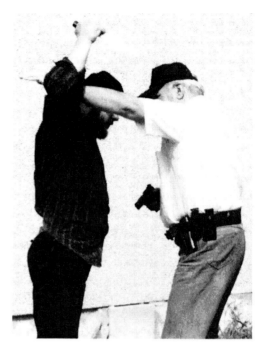

*THE CIRCULAR
SWEEP.*

forearm and open palm of the weak hand, either rotating the arm upward and outward or downward and outward. It is almost an instinctive move, though it should be practiced diligently. The attacker's forearm and weapon are the target, pushing them away from your body. If your enemy has a bladed weapon, you may be slashed in the process, but the wound will most probably be to the outside of the upper arm or forearm—not a very pleasant experience, but much better than a more dangerous cut to your inner forearm, an area filled with nerves and blood vessels. The open palm allows you to grab your adversary's weapon or body, as well as take a knife blow on the palm, again a much better place when compared to a similar slash on the back of the hand.

The object of the exercise is to attempt to deflect your assailant and his weapon away from you while you draw your weapon with your strong hand. Once this is done, an attempt is made to step back and fire your handgun or to assume a proper stance and use your bladed weapon.

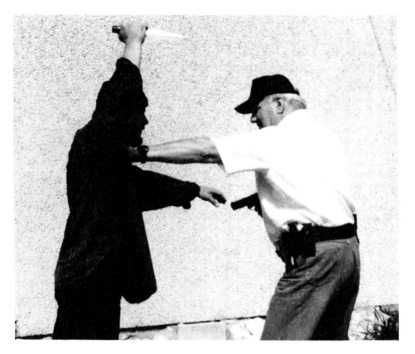

THE PUSH AND STEP BACK.

Another simple and almost instinctive move is to push your armed enemy away from you with the open palm of your weak hand into his chest while you step back, draw your weapon, and then engage him. What you want to achieve is blunting the momentum of his attack, thus throwing him off balance while you seize the initiative.

THOUGHTS ON HANDGUN STOPPING POWER

Probably no subject causes as much controversy in handgunnery than the subject of stopping power. Over the years, I've literally seen otherwise balanced and sane people almost come to blows as they espoused the latest study or theory on the subject.

Without getting into the midst of the battle, let me put forth my thoughts on stopping power.

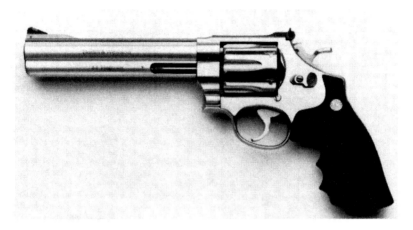

S&W MODEL 629 – CLASSIC: For self-defense with a .44 Magnum, use a 180-grain hollowpoint bullet.

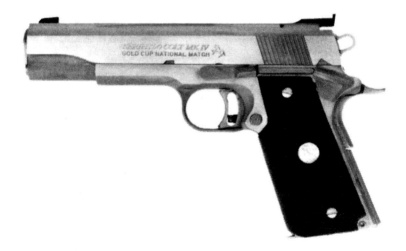

SERIES 80 COLT GOLD CUP MK IV: *An out-of-the-box souped-up Colt for those desiring extra accuracy. NOTE: For heavy field use in mud and sand, it's best to use "loose-as-a-goose" military models for added reliability.*

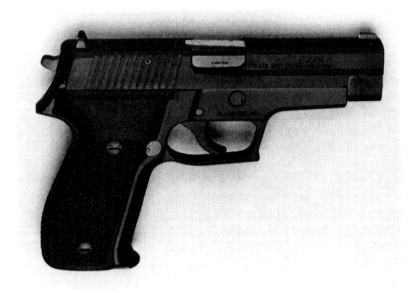

SIG SAUER P226: A large capacity DA auto (15 + 1) that offers state-of-the-art reliability for those desiring a 9mmP handgun.

Bullet Placement
Being able to place a bullet into a critical area of your enemy's anatomy is the main goal. Blowing off your adversary's big toe, while enraging him, will probably not stop him from attempting to continue his attack. We must destroy nerve tissue and/or open up major blood vessels and/or fracture bone used for locomotion. Better still, do all of the above.

Bullet Penetration
For a bullet to do the job it must penetrate deep enough past clothing, skin, muscle, bone, and guts. Superficial wounds may not destroy vital tissue, and the destruction of vital tissue is critical.

Bullet Caliber
The larger the caliber the better chance the bullet has to

destroy vital tissue. The more tissue destroyed, the better. In recent years, the medium calibers (9mmP, .38 Special, .357 Magnum) have been given a needed and vital boost in stopping power by the use of carefully designed bullets that help open them up to big-bore caliber size with regularity. Prior to this, the big-bore calibers (.40, .41, .44, and .45) dominated. Of course, the big boys can be improved to even bigger calibers by the use of the same design magic that allows them to expand without excessive velocity and resultant increased recoil.

Do I Prefer .45 ACP?

Assuming the track through tissue of, for instance, an expanded 9mmP bullet is almost as large as that of an expanded .45 ACP bullet, why would anyone want to carry the heavier .45-caliber bullet? The key word is assume. If the 9mmP doesn't expand, it reacts through tissue just like ball ammo, and the poor track record of the 9mmP was earned by the use of ball ammunition. Second, if I am forced to use ball ammo, I feel much better with the larger wound channel created in tissue by the .45 than the 9mmP.

Bullet placement and magic bullets aside, other factors seem just as important in understanding stopping power. First, the mind-set of the enemy I am shooting at. Fanatics and nut cases are hard to put down with any bullet since they are floating on an adrenaline high. The reason all statistics and studies are controversial is that we do not have any true scientific method of testing bullet stopping power, only empirical ones. We argue over who has the most accurate data, but in reality all data is suspect since, for instance, we cannot even eliminate those who stop on their own accord. Talk to any street cop and he'll tell you of the perp who absorbed a dozen supposedly lethal shots, continued to run around firing his weapon, and lived. Then he'll tell you the story of the guy who was shot in the arm, dropped his gun, and sat down and died from fear.

A second factor that is hardly ever discussed is the mind-set of the guy firing the manstopper bullet. Having confidence in one's handgun and choice of bullet, coupled with good training technique, goes a long way in assuring that our bullets will get into our enemy's boiler room and shut him down. Never carry a weapon/ammo combo that you do not feel absolutely confident with. The performance of the good guy is important to that critical first-shot placement and then with those follow-up shots.

A third factor, one which we have a hard time controlling, is luck. We may think we hit the exact physical location we were aiming for, but we do not see the desired result. Why? Maybe the bullet only nicked that artery or bone. Maybe it hit nerve tissue but did not really disrupt it. Lady Luck is still a factor to be contended with in stopping power.

I would not lose any sleep if I were forced to use 9mmP in any form, since bullet placement is still the key to stopping power, and I feel confident in placing most of my shots correctly. However, for my most comfortable mind-set and from my reading of the data, I still prefer to strap a brace of .45s on.

The medium calibers are debated about. Maybe they work, maybe they have been vastly improved. Then again, maybe not. It is still very controversial. When it comes to survival, I try to avoid controversy and debate whenever possible. Street survival needs all the help it can get; every little bit helps. In the final analysis, that little bit more confidence and caliber provided by the time-proven .45 suits me just fine.

Case Study: Attack of the Sudani

In October of 1953, thousands of Arab terrorists, then called Fedeyeen, were stationed in the Gaza Strip, which at that time was under the control of Egypt, which had captured it in Israel's 1948 War of Independence. Egyptian intelligence paid them for crossing the border. Their mission? To place mines along the roads of southern Israel and cause as many civilian casualties as possible. Arik Sharon, Schlomo Baum, and some commandos of the elite unit 101 were ordered into the area and, on the successful completion of their mission of attacking a terrorist base, moved back through the desert toward the Israeli border. Only the light of a thin crescent desert moon lit the way. All seemed to be going well, when suddenly a squad of Sudanese soldiers ("Sudani" in Hebrew) who were allied with the Egyptians charged at them.

Baum opened up with his Tommy gun and the Sudani jumped to the side of the path. All except one. A big, tall fellow who was the leader charged on.

E.S.: What was he armed with?

S.B.: A rifle. When he raised it, I fired a burst which hit him. One good thing about the .45 bullet at night—you can hear it smack into a human target with a very distinctive sound. The 9mmP doesn't make this sound. So those three loud smacks told me I had connected three times, though of course I did not know exactly where he was hit.

E.S.: Did he go down?

S.B.: No. I distinctly remember three occasions when the big .45 bullet did not result in an instant stop. This was one of those times. No cartridge can do that 100 percent of the time. That's why you must have enough ammo on you to continue the battle until your enemy or enemies do go down forever. Incidentally, in later raids we carried 9mmP German Schmeissers (the lighter weapon and bullets were easier to carry on long marches). The 9mmP was not as decisive a manstopper as the .45 ACP but was adequate.

E.S.: You mentioned he didn't go down. What happened?

S.B.: He kept on charging at me as if nothing had happened. I squeezed the trigger, and all I heard was a click; the magazine was empty. He would be on me in another split second. I had no time to change magazines. I instantly decided to use surprise.

E.S.: Surprise?

S.B.: I shouted at him in Arabic: "Wait a moment!" He stopped dead in his tracks, so confused he didn't shoot.

E.S.: What did you do then?

S.B.: The unexpected. I slammed him over the head with the full weight of that Tommy gun. I was young and strong then, able to kill a donkey with one blow of my fist to its head. He crashed down, dead before he hit the ground. The next Israeli commando who followed sprayed the other Sudani down good, and we charged past them and out into open desert.

··

STREET SURVIVAL LESSONS

1) *Warding off an attacker.* The circular sweep block and the push and step back block are effective and easy to learn.

2) *Nothing stops an enemy 100-percent of the time.* Never believe any projectile gives 100-percent stops, not even with multiple shots.

3) *High capacity.* Within the limits of weapon control and portability, high capacity has its place.

4) *Use surprise.* Surprise is a good tactic. Use it. Yell. Distract. It may just work.

5) *Innovate.* The stopping power of a Tommy gun delivered over the head is a most excellent fight-stopper.

··

THE LONG GUN

Carrying a rifle, submachine gun, or shotgun as a street survival weapon may seem an unlikely possibility in some parts of the globe. Certainly, I have never seen anyone walking on Wilshire Boulevard in Los Angeles with an M16 in hand. I have seen this in Israel; in fact, it is a common occurrence here, as in many other nations. Tens of thousands of Israeli settlers, soldiers, and Border Police (quasi-military police units) fill the streets here, and no one gives their long guns a thought. It is part of the landscape. It is not uncommon for Israeli civilians, coming from isolated places and set-

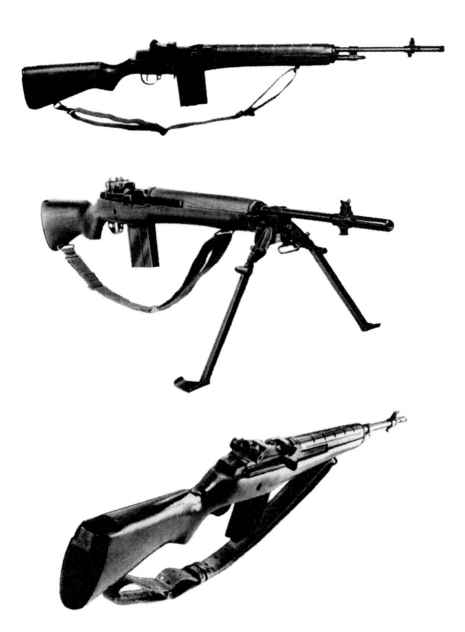

SPRINGFIELD ARMORY M1A RIFLE: A quality copy of the battle-proven M14.

tlements, to be armed with Uzis and M1 Carbines, openly displayed and carried. These weapons are not privately owned (Israel suffers from many gun laws, which forbid rifle ownership for all except .22 LR caliber, a legacy of the British Mandatory Period) but rather are checked out of a village or settlement arms room. For example, I have a very accurate M14 rifle with 3X-9X telescope, which I keep in my bedroom, ready for instant use. I checked it out of my settlement arms room to fulfill my role as the settlement sniper. I also checked out an M1 Carbine, loading its magazines with Winchester 110-grain jacketed hollowpoints.

I have always been partial to the M14, considering it the finest battle rifle ever, bar none, and I was instrumental in getting one into each Israeli rifle squad for the squad sniper.

I like a weapon that can reach out there and still be excellent for close-quarter combat. Nothing points as well for point shooting as a good, full-power battle rifle. Yes, you heard me right—for point fire, or, as some call it, "instinctive fire."

The Battle Rifle

The ideal battle rifle (and street and survival weapon) is a semiautomatic full-powered (7.62mm NATO caliber) weapon that can reach out to 1,000 yards and hit a human target and still have the capability of engaging multiple aggressors at almost contact range without the use of sights. I believe no other standard-production military rifle fills the bill as well as the M14.

Live-Fire Demonstration at Mitzpeh Ramon

Mitzpeh Ramon is located in the Negev desert in southern Israel and is part of the great Quatara Depression, a Grand Canyon-like crack in the earth that runs from Syria to Africa. It is a rather sparsely settled part of the country and was the site of a new sniper course I was supervising. We were standing on a high desert plateau when the helicopter of then Chief of Staff Gen. Raful Eitan landed. He was coming to inspect the setup and facilities of the new sniper course.

Never one to miss an opportunity to make a pitch for

some of the ideas created at the World Institute (the Jerusalem-based think tank where I worked with Baum in its military section), I pushed for a demonstration of my ideas on point fire with the sniper rifle.

Another idea I created was The Uniform Shooting

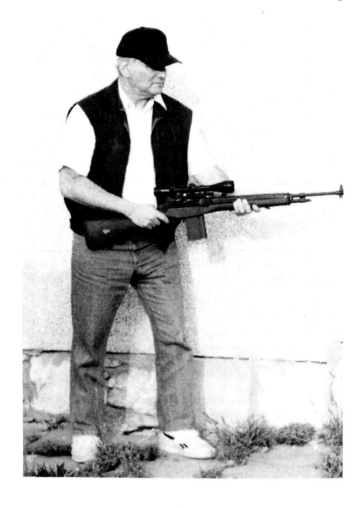

SNIPER RIFLE POINT-FIRED FROM THE HIP: Even a scoped sniper rifle can be point-fired from the hip. Over the telescope, quick fire also works.

System—a multiweapon training system based on the unique concept that all hand-held projectile launchers, such as pistols, submachine guns, carbines, rifles, shotguns, and shoulder-fired rockets are really the same. This somewhat different mind-set allows uniform training methods to be devised that are most cost-effective and battle-efficient. For example, point fire is point fire no matter what the hand-held launcher looks like, a revolutionary concept at the time.

With this in mind, I decided to put on a live-fire demonstration using the fine Israeli Sirkiss M-26 Sniper Rifle, a 7.62mm NATO-caliber semiauto based on the battle-proven AK-47 design. At the time, I was pushing hard for what I and Baum called a "battle sniper" (sharpshooter) in each squad and then a squad of more conventional two-man sniper teams at battalion. (We settled on the title battle sniper for the squad sniper, and it is now standard in the Israel Defense Forces.) There had been a move to bring a bolt-action rifle into service, and I was dead-set against the idea, considering it dangerous to the sniper in today's modern and fluid battlefield. Only a semiauto would do. Now you may legitimately ask, what has this to do with street survival? My answer is everything.

I set up two man-size targets and spread them about a half yard apart. Standing facing them, I proceeded to fire a single bullet into each one in turn, moving ever backward, blowing out chunks of target up to about the 30-yard line. All this with unsighted point fire. The Lord was good to me that day—I didn't miss even once. The General turned to me with more than just a little surprise and asked, "Can you teach soldiers to do that?"

I assured him I could and stressed that this could only be done with a semiauto rifle and that was why our snipers needed such a semiautomatic weapon and not a bolt action.

Unfortunately, the Sirkiss rifle never made it into official service, fine weapon though it was, but one resembling it did. It was based on the Israeli Galil in 7.62mm NATO. I do not believe this rifle is as good as the almost handmade Sirkiss M26 sniper rifle. I had originally wanted the American M21, but since that was not available, we settled for handpicked M14s. I pushed for us to purchase them after the United States made the monumental error of selling them off to the world at the ridiculous cost of $10 apiece, including spare parts. (At least the ones bought by Israel got into the hands of a staunch U.S. ally.) Israel now had battle snipers who could function in the midst of combat and not only along its periphery. The complete battle sniper was born.

Long Guns for Street Survival

Even if you live in a part of the world where the open carry of long guns is not the norm, it would still seem very prudent to have such weapons and know how to use them just in case the worst-case scenarios in this unsettled and uncertain world come to fruition.

The use of these weapons in the street may entail their use at contact or close-to-contact distance. For too long we have focused on battle rifles as being "teachers," assault rifles as being upgraded submachine guns, submachine guns as being "sprayers," carbines as being upgraded pistols, and shotguns as being "scatterguns." We sometimes forget that these uses may not be the only way to incorporate them into our street survival arsenal, where close-quarter combat is the overwhelming order of the day (unless we are facing a full-blown civil insurrection or worse). Point shooting is the king of street survival with firearms, since most deadly confrontations of a criminal nature take place at a distance of 1 to 3 meters and in bad light.

UNIFORM SHOOTING SYSTEM: POINT SHOOTING

Look upon the firearm in your hand as a launcher and not just as a pistol or rifle, etc. What you want to do is simple and easy. You want to point that launcher at a target or targets and have it launch a deadly projectile into your enemy or enemies so that they cease and desist aggressive action. You want to be able to do this with single or multiple targets, at ranges from contact distance to 3 yards or more (point: hip

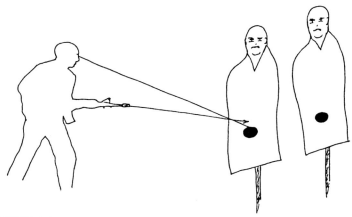

QUICK-FIRE TRAINING TARGETS.

fire) and up to 30 yards plus (point: quick fire) as a maximum, knowing that the contact-distance-to-7-yard figure is the much more important distance in unsighted fire. Beyond that, sighted fire is usually possible, though one should still be able to use point: quick fire if needed.

To become proficient in point shooting, set two man-sized targets up at 1 yard and have them be about 1/2-yard apart and in line. Have a human face staring at you from the target. Always do this, as it conditions you to what your target really is—a man. Place a bright red circle about 6 inches in diameter directly below and in line with the belly button of each target. For practice, a white line (tape or thin white wooden strip) can be placed on top of any weapon you have, be it a pistol, rifle, shotgun, etc., so that you have a clear sighting plane that you can pick up with peripheral vision. The use of the white line is not mandatory, but it helps. So do the circles that are placed low. Why? Most people shoot over their targets. This helps you to focus at something near to but below the midline of your enemy. Why two targets? Because we tend to keep repeating shooting mistakes in point fire, and the use of two targets helps us to break our pattern and correct any mistakes as we fire. (A useful by-product is that it conditions the mind to engage multiple targets.)

When learning something new, never try for lightning speed. Speed is simply a by-product of diligent and persistent training and not a way to train, at least at first. I used to tell my students, "Do it slowly and well. I don't want you to be the fastest man in the graveyard. Speed will come later."

Face the targets and draw your holstered pistol *slowly*, pointing it at the red circle with one hand. Use two hands with your "long guns." (In a later exercise you can attempt one-handed point shooting if said long guns are light enough for this task. This is only for emergency use.)

Point Fire: Hip Shooting (1 to 3 Yards)

By using point fire (hip shooting) and not looking at the sights but at that red circle, fire one bullet at the left target, two at the right one, and one back to the left one. I have recently added the point fire double tap to the right target. Why? Because in multiple target exercises you should always fire single bullets into each target in line until you engage the last one, double tap this one, and then fire a bullet into each of the previously engaged targets as you shoot them back down the line.

Uniformity and repetition are what the motor system of the brain likes best when learning technique. Never train one way and then expect to perform another way under stress. While some things are instinctive (crouching under fire and the convulsive grip), most other things have to be learned and imprinted deep into our psyche.

Our goal is to hit both targets 100 percent (military standards are 3 out of 4 shots because of the cost problems inherent in mass training). When we are able to do this, we step back to the 2-yard line and repeat the exercise. This is done again at the 3-yard line. This is unsighted point fire at the contact-to-3-yard range (hip shooting).

Point Shooting: Quick Fire (3 to 30 Yards)

From contact distance to 3 yards, hip shooting works well for the average shooter. When the distance widens beyond 3 yards, we should have sufficient time to bring the weapon up to below eye level and, aiming above the sights, shoot at the enemy by a type of point shooting called quick fire. In this system, the isosceles two-handed hold seems to work with the pistol, though once again you may only be able to use one hand. Your long weapon will have to be held in two hands, since raising it to such a level with one hand leads to instability and loss of control, unless you are a hero of a Hollywood film, where such feats are commonplace.

Beyond 7 yards, you may have enough time to use the sights, though true aimed fire still may be difficult. With the long gun I have seen good work done in quick fire out to and

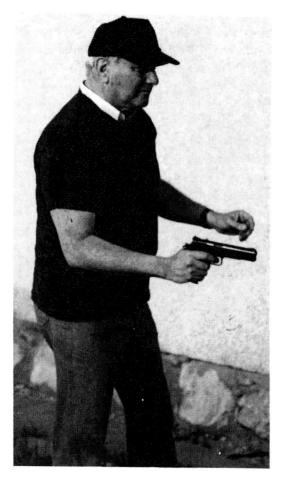

POINT—HIP FIRE: *At really close quarters, point-fire hip shooting with one hand should be an emergency option.*

beyond 30 yards, though once again, aimed fire is preferred.

Beyond 30 yards, maybe even 15 yards, sighted fire is more accurate for many shooters, and the Weaver hold for the pistol becomes ideal. Remember, we are not speaking of absolutes. Variations and changes can be made. For example, the Weaver or isosceles hold can be chosen for any position; the choice is yours. Stick with one if you prefer. I quizzed Baum about this.

E.S.: At what range can unaimed fire (without conventional sights) be used?

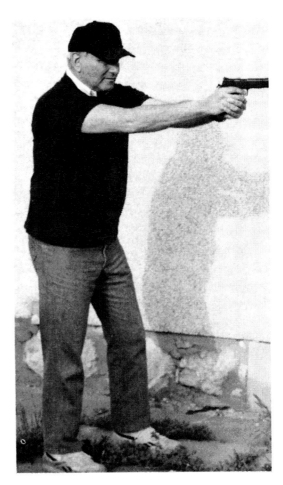

POINT—QUICK FIRE: As the distance increases, one may have time to use two hands in the isosceles hold. The convulsive grip and instinctive crouch are used since this is more natural when your enemy is still close. NOTE: Weaver hold also works if you train for it.

S.B.: I have never made a study of the subject, but in Commando 101 we were able to put a burst of full-automatic fire into the window of a building at 100 meters without the use of sights. Of course, this was during daylight hours, and we had the added help of seeing our bullets hit dry ground in front of the target. Correcting our stream of bullets was therefore quite simple.

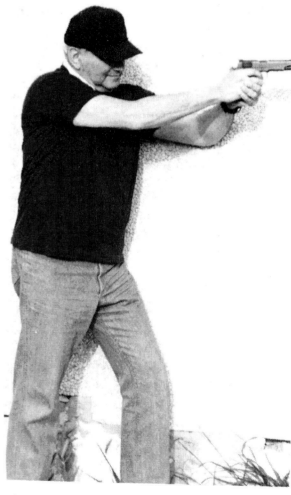

AIMED FIRE: When your adversary is at longer ranges, the use of the two-handed Weaver hold and sights is ideal. NOTE: Some claim only one system (Weaver, isosceles, etc.) should be used. I disagree. For example, one learns many shooting positions (standing, kneeling, prone) so as to best handle a particular situation. I like the option of knowing more than one system. Use what works best for you. Hit the target. That's what really counts in the end.

However, we had an unlimited ammunition supply, literally truckloads full. That's what made the feat so simple. Practice, practice, and more practice until we could place that stream of bullets just about anywhere we wanted. It may seem like a stunt, but in a firefight it's important to have all these skills. One never knows the situation one can find oneself in.

E.S: What type of rifles, submachine guns, and shotguns do you recommend for "alley cleaning"?

S.B.: I've always preferred semiautomatic and full-automatic systems in all weapons with as large a capacity as possible. Caliber is important, but I'm still partial to lots of bullets that are already in the gun. Within reason, high capacity is more important to me than that slightly heavier caliber. I can live with 9mmP in my pistols and submachine guns and 5.56mm in my rifles over the larger .45 ACP and 7.62mm NATO calibers. Life sometimes is a compromise. That's mine. Shotguns are not my forté.

SHOTGUNS

Baum, like many Israelis and Europeans, is not familiar with shotgun use for close-quarter firefights. This is probably due to the ready availability of Uzis for this task. Personally, I find shotguns suited for street survival as long as the distances involved aren't much over 40 yards. The caliber of choice is 12 gauge, and 00 or #4 buck (if available) is the best shell to put into the gun. I prefer semiauto shotguns. I do not like pump shotguns because they necessitate the use of two hands to load each shell into its chamber mechanically, a really Herculean task when wrestling with some hothead in the street.

I also find that pump actions are difficult to work when one is lying flat in the street. Keep them for sporting use. For street survival, use a semiauto. These shotguns can even be shot one-handed in a pinch. I find these attributes of the semiauto too important to be cast aside for the familiarity of that pump shotgun in your closet.

As far as caliber is concerned, I disagree with Baum in his choice of 9mmP over the .45 ACP. Caliber is important in street survival. You need all the edge you can muster up in a close-quarter encounter. Baum is a former commando who tracked dozens of miles in reprisal raids into enemy territory. For that, the lighter weight of the 9mmP submachine gun and ammunition, plus the added capacity, was a major factor to be considered. I don't see this as a major factor in street survival.

In the rifle category, caliber is less critical, though I still like the capability of the 7.62mm NATO cartridge over the 5.56mm. It has the ability to breech cover more decisively and the added plus of being able to reach out way beyond the range of the 5.56mm. I like the 5.56mm, though, and wouldn't lose any sleep if restricted to it for inner city use.

SUBMACHINE GUNS

I am not a fan of submachine guns used only in the full-auto mode, considering this to be a waste of precious ammo. I do see submachine guns as weapons that, like shotguns, are special weapons for special situations, e.g., for cleaning antagonists out of close-quarter environments such as trenches or rooms or for blunting a sudden close-quarter mass attack by many, such as a mob of berserk rioters.

William, a close friend and ex-paratrooper, does not agree, putting my negative feelings about full-auto fire down to age. He claims many people over 50 years of age think the same way, preferring aimed, single-shot fire to burst fire. He has a case to prove his point.

Case Study: Shots in the Dark

William carries his Uzi with a heavy-duty flashlight tied to its front stock, the flashlight being activated by touching a pressure switch. He keeps the gun on full auto when he moves in what he considers are dangerous conditions, which is just about all the time.

Driving through a village one dark night with another

Israeli at the wheel, they found themselves the unwilling recipients of a shower of heavy rocks, iron bars, and slabs of concrete thrown from the rooftops of buildings bordering a narrow street.

E.S.: Could you drive away?

W: Not easily. They had laid obstacles in the road that not only blocked most of it but also forced us to slow down and move in the direction they wanted, which was closer to the buildings. They knew what they were doing.

E.S.: How many of them were there?

W: I guesstimated about 20 to 30. It was hard seeing them since they ran to the edge of the roofs, attacked us, and then melted away. I'll tell you one thing, it was a real tense situation. It sounded like a thousand hail storms all rolled into one. The front window of the pickup was shattered, and the roof caved in like it was made of cardboard. I got glass in my eyes—bad luck, as this was the first time I forgot to wear my clear shooting glasses, which I always do when driving.

E.S.: Murphy's Law.

W: Exactly. Sort of like the new police officer who was assigned to me and who forgot his bullet-resistant vest. He was shot, survived, and practically lived in it after that. I almost lost an eye because I forgot those glasses. I'll never forget them again.

E.S.: What did you do next?

W: We debussed and, using the pickup as cover, went on the offensive. It wasn't long before two of them charged at me with Molotov cocktails, coming up a dark alley between two buildings.

The fire from the Molotovs helped me spot them. I pressed the pressure switch and they were caught in the beam of the flashlight. I fired a long burst (I meant to fire short, controlled ones), and they went down like a ton of bricks.

E.S.: Dead?

W: I didn't wait around to see, but I think so, since they lay with their legs crossed all funny-like, something I've seen before out on the street—usually a sign of death.

We jumped back into the pickup and slowly weaved through the dark, this time firing short bursts, and some not so short, at the tops of the buildings where dark figures wildly pranced around throwing debris down on us. When we got to the end of the street, another one ran toward us with a blazing Molotov. I fired and he went down the same way. My buddy says he thinks he winged another one. We finally got through in a truck that looked like it was in World War II. I mean it was totaled. My buddy was pissed as hell, but we got out of it in one piece.

E.S.: What did you do then?

W: I reported what happened to some Israelis manning a roadblock. They looked like security people. One glance at our vehicle convinced them it was a justifiable shooting. We went back to look over the area with them, but an eerie silence and darkness was all that we saw or heard.

E.S.: What about the ones you shot?

W: Not a sign of them, but as you know they don't like to leave their dead around because they know we have to do autopsies on them. They don't like autopsies.

STREET SURVIVAL LESSONS

1) *Full-auto fire works.* Modern submachine guns can accurately blanket an area with a long burst of full-auto fire, though shorter, controlled bursts are preferred in order to save ammo.

2) *Gun-mounted flashlight.* The use of a flashlight that has a pressure-activated switch seems to have saved the day for William and his friend since it framed the perpetrators in bright light and acted as an effective night vision sight. Of course, only put the light on at the instant of fire, since it also acts as a beacon for return enemy fire.

3) *De-bus when under attack.* Sitting in the pickup

would have given them narrowed vision and less chance to respond to close-quarter attack. It would have also limited their field of fire. If those burning Molotov cocktails had splashed into the pickup, the story would have turned out quite differently.

FIREARMS SAFETY

I present the following to Israelis in my lectures:

a) Before you handle any gun, you must learn how it operates and how to put it in a safe condition.

b) Treat every gun as if it were loaded, even after you (or anyone) have unloaded it and know it is unloaded.

c) As soon as you pick up a gun, open its action and inspect it to see if it is loaded.

d) Be sure the gun barrel is clear of obstructions before you fire it on the shooting range.

e) Never keep a gun loaded when it is being stored.

f) Never point a gun at anyone you do not intend to shoot.

g) Avoid ricochet. Never fire at a flat surface or water.

h) Store guns and ammo separately and out of the reach of children.

i) Alcohol and guns don't mix.

j) Do not play with guns.

k) Concentrate. Do not let your attention wander when you are holding a gun.

l) Guns are dangerous. They are never to be handled by anyone without your express permission.

m) Unloading a double-action revolver: All you have to do to render the gun safe is to swing its cylinder out. Then unload it.

n) Unloading a semiauto pistol: Remove its magazine first and then put the magazine into your pocket. Keep your finger off the trigger and then use the free hand to pull the slide

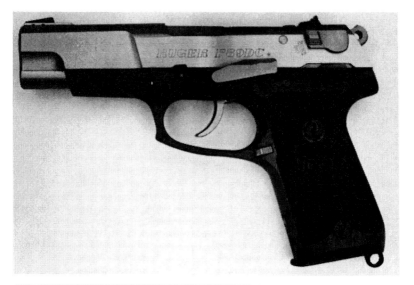

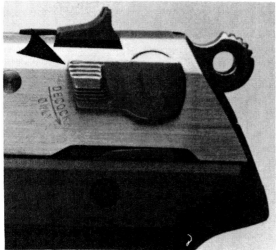

RUGER DECOCKER PISTOL: While built-in safety helps cut down on gun accidents, nothing can be substituted for the shooter's vigilance.

back and lock it, allowing the chamber to be inspected. Unless you ejected a cartridge, put your finger against the barrel chamber to feel if the round is really out. If a live round is in the chamber, remove it.

PRINCIPLE OF UNIFORMITY:
LOADING AND UNLOADING A FIREARM

Avoiding tragic death or accidents begins with your attitude toward firearms safety. The rule of uniformity can help you if you strictly adhere to it. Always make the loading or unloading of your guns as well as your means of storage into a routine procedure. Try to do these tasks in the same place and in the same manner. Always concentrate on the job at hand and not, for example, on the antics of your fellow police officers in the locker room or your kids at home. It is very hard to concentrate on two things at once. When firearms are one of these things, the results can be tragic. Only think, see, and do the job at hand when handling firearms. Try never to vary the routine and, if possible, try to do these tasks when you are alone and without any outside distractions. A bullet, once launched, can't be called back.

Chapter Five

Guns Rigs
for the Street

Those of us working as professionals in the field of street survival must be aware of history. The history of the Wild West gunslinger has much to teach us. One man stands out. That man is John Wesley Hardin. Hardin was an unreconstructed rebel who was a born gunslinger, killing his first man while still in his teens. In no time, Hardin became a seasoned killer, shooting a bloody trail across the North American continent. He was a man who lived by the gun. A criminal, but a very special one.

We can say something in his favor. He did have one idiosyncrasy that was quite rare for most of his ilk: he prided himself on always giving his enemies a fighting chance. Of course, this really wasn't much of a chance, since Hardin was so superior to anyone around. Still, his attitude was a refreshing change from the back-shooting technique favored by just about everyone.

Hardin's superiority was based on endless practice and a scientific evaluation of each detail of what made up a gunfight. It was also based on the fact that he was absolutely cold and ruthless in a most professional manner when engaging in deadly combat. He was a student of the art of killing. Hardin sometimes carried a leather vest that had two holsters sewn into it. They carried his brace of matching six-guns in the front cavalry draw position, butts forward. This is, to my mind, a most excellent manner in which to carry a brace of pistols—lightning fast and instantly available to either hand.

The system did have one problem: unless you wore a loose-fitting jacket or coat, the pistols could be seen—not a big problem in Hardin's time but a definite minus in ours. Hardin was killed by a peace officer named John Selman, who brought him down the only way anyone knew how, with a shot to the back.

Hardin, the greatest gunfighter of them all, died in El Paso, Texas, on August 19, 1895.

MY RIG: A VARIATION OF HARDIN'S

I've always felt that studying such men was an excellent way of broadening one's horizons. Knowing that Hardin's system was not totally useful for my needs, I made a belt-carry variation of his technique. I now carry two Colt 1911s, two Lightweight Commanders, or two Star PDs in front cross draw rigs, butts forward, finding them fast on the draw, most concealable with a little know-how, and, best of all, applicable for instant use by either hand so as to cover all worst-case scenarios. I remain convinced that John Wesley Hardin knew what gunslinging was all about.

This was brought to my mind in a recent shooting contest I took part in out in the "West Bank." I succeeded in out-drawing my compatriots and puncturing my target with just enough of an edge to win. I learned that fast draw is not only based on speed (time) but on distance. In actuality, I drew more slowly than some of the others, but the distance my hand traveled was shorter.

Studying all manner of attacks by street scum has convinced me that one's primary and secondary handgun must be available for instant use by either hand. That and studying

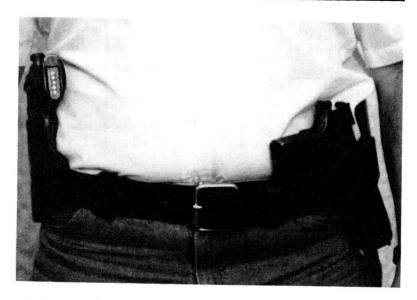

MY RIG: A variation of John Wesley Hardin's design, allowing a brace of pistols to be drawn by either hand. For comfort, I've come to prefer the weak-handed holster tilted more vertically than the strong-handed one.

Hardin were the reasons I dropped the strong-side so-called FBI carry (featured in my Paladin Press video, *Secrets of Gunfighting Israeli Style*) and moved my backup handgun forward to the left-handed front cross draw position.

I now carry my brace of matching .45 autos in the right and left front draw positions. I repeat, this idea is not new. I have just refined it to fit my personal needs. It just might suit your needs, too.

Under an Open Jacket or Vest

Concealment under an open jacket or vest allows for much leeway in the size of the weapons carried in that the standard grips of the 1911s pose no concealment problem. The weight of the jacket or vest can, of course, vary with the season, and one can today find these items made of very light material if desired for summer use. I have found it to be fastest of all concealment setups.

The belt rig can be placed onto the gun belt holding your pants up (I only use gun belts for this chore and find two of them work nicely for both tasks), and then both are secured by belt keepers.

One can also simply put both holsters and magazine pouches directly onto the gun belt holding the trousers up. I, like many police officers, find the single gun belt technique very tiring in that everything on it must be removed at the end of the day.

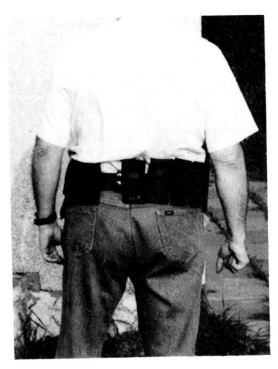

LOADED MAGAZINE FOR EITHER HAND:
Keep magazines on both sides of the body so that either hand can easily grab one in an emergency.

That's why I like the second over-belt setup so much more.

Winter Variation

I have used this idea in the winter with a small variation. The second over gun belt is simply placed over the sweatshirt or sweater, resting on top of the gun belt underneath. This is very comfortable and easy to get on and off. Actually, I've even tried this variation by placing the gun rig onto the top of the gun belt holding up the pants and found it to work very well in that here again, I did not need to use belt keepers.

Belt Holster and Fanny Pack

For hot weather, I have come up with an idea that works very well where carrying one gun openly is socially acceptable, but not two. I use a left front draw holster for a .45 auto and put another in a fanny pack. The holster is on a second gun belt that is placed over my pant gun belt, and the fanny pack is placed over this. All is held together by belt keepers. This is a secure rig.

Double Belly Band

A useful variation of this setup is the use of two belly band holsters, one over the other, when high concealment is necessary. This setup hides nicely under a sweater, shirt, or even T-shirt. The handguns and any magazines are carried in the same general area of the anatomy, as are the guns carried on the belt. The principle of uniformity has not been breached.

This type of gun carry is, however, a little slower in getting your guns in hand, though leaving some shirt buttons open can help improve this. Sewing false buttons on your shirt (making it look closed) while fitting Velcro snaps in

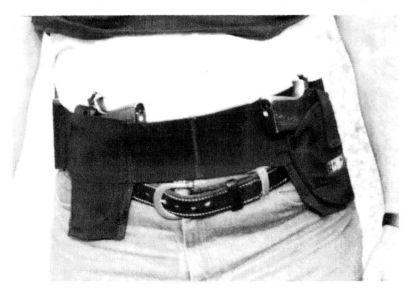

DOUBLE BELLY BAND RIG.

their place is certainly better than having to undo buttons, though one could simply rip the shirt open in an emergency. Problem is, this can be hard on shirts if you are a stickler for real-life training scenarios.

I have some good news for those guys who are, shall we say, heavily endowed with adipose tissue around the gut. Place the belly band higher up the chest rather than at belt level, where it is usually extremely uncomfortable for some. The shape of this area tends to hold the bands as solid as the rock of Gibraltar, almost turning them into a double shoulder holster rig.

The principle of uniformity is not violated if you keep the handguns in the general body area of your belt carry—once again, a compromise, this time for concealability, but not a deadly compromise. It works out on the street. I use the system with a brace of matching Star PDs.

Under Clothing

Concealing either rig under an outside garment means wearing a light shirt or undershirt between the gun rig and your skin. To do otherwise will result in discomfort caused by chafing or sweating. Make sure the overgarment can be easily lifted or opened by the weak hand if necessary and allows enough room for a reasonably fast draw with either hand.

Handgun Backup to a Long Gun

When I carry a handgun as a backup to a rifle, submachine gun, or shotgun, I have found that the variation of Hardin's carry works very well for me. The front cross system keeps the long gun far enough away that it doesn't get tangled up in shooting or when carried in a rifle strap strung on the shoulder (during the rare times I use rifle straps; I find I can get my rifle to shoulder much faster without one). I have found the Hardin variation rig far superior to having a handgun in a high-ride-carry holster on the side the rifle calls home, an idea that any hunter of man or beast will probably agree with. In the FBI carry, your long gun will pound against your handgun, beating both items up in short order.

Besides being very uncomfortable and inefficient, it makes noise, telegraphing your presence. The strong-side carry does work well if you are on horseback. Wearing the handgun in this area, but further back toward the kidneys, is comfortable. This is all the more so if the long gun is kept in a sheath tied to the saddle. Alas, this becomes mere nostalgia for most, since such methods of transportation are not the general rule in our world. Today, most use jeeps to roam around in. In a vehicle, the strong-side FBI high-ride carry will jam into the rear seat and back into your back unless it is carried in front of the hip bone. Fitting the holster or holsters to our individual needs is vital. For my needs, my variation of Hardin's double front cross draw position works very well, even with a rifle or carbine in hand or on the right shoulder.

HOW MUCH AMMO?

A question that keeps popping up from my readers and students is "How much ammo is enough?" My standard reply is that I have never heard of anyone dying from having too much ammo on him, only from too much ammo in him. Having more than enough ammunition for any altercation is the goal. Knowing that more than enough ready ammunition is on one's person has a very profound and beneficial effect on one's psychological outlook and helps boost one's ego. This is not to say one may waste ammunition. I have always believed that frugality in ammunition expenditure is a definite plus.

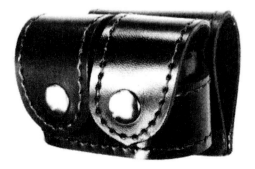

SAFARILAND DOUBLE SPEED-LOADER POUCH. With the revolver, one can never have too many of these filled with cartridges and ready for instant action.

Make each bullet count and call your shots. Spraying precious ammo around the landscape in a gunfight is stupid and can get one quite killed if carried to the extreme.

I set off my gun rig with eight loaded magazines on my gun belt (this is a change from the past, when six was my standard), all to the sides of the hip and rear. My 60-round minimum of major-caliber handgun ammo is never breached. This means I never count the ammo for a third or fourth handgun in the 60-round minimum. All such rounds (like handguns) are considered extra.

If I carry a long gun, I consider 90 rounds of ammo to be in the ballpark as a minimum figure and try to increase that amount if going into isolated areas of the country. I have found such a minimum gives me solid worst-case-scenario answers.

AMMUNITION UNIFORMITY

The principle of uniformity must not be breached even with the type of ammunition we choose for the street. Keeping a magazine filled with ultra-high-penetrating ammo for the highway and low-penetrating for the shopping mall is a very difficult thing to juggle in one's mind when the chips are down. Of course, one can be trained to automatically remember to change magazines as conditions vary, but is it all worth it for most of us? I have found that regular military .45 ACP ball ammo, as well as all 230-grain hollowpoint loads, penetrate today's cars very well. Why complicate matters more than one needs to? Working on the problem has convinced me that I do not need special magazines for extremely special-purpose ammo. Unless you are in the SWAT business or some such specialty line of work where such ammo might be called for, my recommendation is to keep it simple.

Tactical Reload
Another idea I challenge is the so-called tactical reload, where a partially filled magazine is changed for a filled one instead of letting the magazine run dry in a firefight. This is okay for a SWAT team about to charge, but not for everyone else.

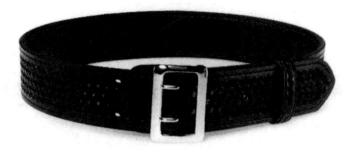

SAFARILAND GUN BELT.

The practice can lead to confusion in a gunfight. I know it is popular in IPSC competition, but that's competition. Out on the street, jamming your partially fired magazines back into your magazine pouches is a mistake for almost all survival scenarios except for the valiant charge at an enemy position. I have seen some trainers tell students to place partially fired magazines in this and that place on the gun belt, seemingly believing that anyone should be able to remember which magazines are which in a real gunfight. Maybe you can, maybe they can, but I'll tell you something—I can't. I believe in the rule "keep it simple."

BUY QUALITY

We have all seen the guy in the gun store who buys what is considered the top-quality state-of-the-art handgun and then shops around for a cheap holster and belt to carry it in. You should choose street accessories and accouterments with the same mind-set and care as anything you stake your life on. Economize on that trip you wanted to take next year, not on what you carry in the street. There is no economy class in street survival.

Whatever alterations to holsters and other equipment I have written about for my personal carry needs I have always done on first-line equipment that did not quite suit a particular need I envisioned. I experiment with and carry only quality items.

The Gun Belt

When wearing a gun belt, you should try to have it at least 1 inch wide and a 1/4 inch thick for handguns weighing in under about 25 ounces. A 1 1/2-inch belt and up of the same thickness is recommended for all handguns weighing in at 26 ounces or higher. Wear your belt tight enough so that your thumb, if slid between your body and the gun butt, will move the gun butt back, pressing it into your body. There is nothing more uncomfortable and detrimental to daily wear in the street than ill-fitting carry equipment. Discomfort leads to constant shifting or taking equipment off, both extremely bad habits.

RIG TRICKS

Being, by nature, a constant experimenter when it comes to street survival, I have put forward some ideas in this book that have been street-proven for more than 40 years. I do not base this just on interviewing those who work out there but on personal experience in actually testing each and every idea over and over in every type of climatic and social condition. Though most everything has been settled on, I still find each day a learning process where new ideas are tested and old ones reevaluated.

Waist-High Uniformity

The principle of uniformity is alive and well and just as important when you carry accessories and accouterments. Reaching for a nonexistent gun magazine or backup knife can be extremely disconcerting in a tight situation. We are only speaking of seconds, maybe even milliseconds, but time can work against you in a most unfortunate manner when your life is at stake.

Personally, I prefer to carry everything needed for street survival at waistband height. Human hands are in that general vicinity most of the time and shouldn't have far to go when that speed loader or magazine is needed. For ultimate uniformity under stress, the same general area of the body should have each item needed. Ideally, each item should be in exactly the same place and in exactly the same kind of carrier, though this is not always feasible. Compromises, as long as the general body area rule is adhered to, can be made. When working the farm, I wear a light overshirt in summertime or a jacket over this in winter to keep the elements out and the shock of all that hardware from the eyes of visitors when I go to the front gate.

Belt Magazine Pouches

My variation of Hardin's setup uses a leather gun belt with two open IPSC-type plastic holders for .45 magazines and six synthetic material magazine flap pouches. The main thing is that holsters and magazines are in the same general area of the body in all setups.

What is bad about those skimpy IPSC plastic magazine holders is that they will throw their magazines out and over the landscape at the first opportunity, such as when you're wrestling with a perp or bouncing in an open jeep. What is good about them is that they are fast for getting magazine in hand.

I am keenly aware of the lack of rough usage capability of these IPSC holders and carry them only because I have six more magazines on me that are much more resistant to losing their contents. That's many more than most of the peo-

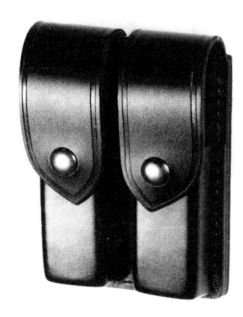

SAFARILAND DOUBLE MAGAZINE

ple I know carry, and that's my minimum, not my maximum. I can afford to sacrifice retention for speed with those first two magazines in that I also carry a matching backup gun, the fastest reload around. I have used this combination for years and do not seem inclined to change it, even after much experimentation and testing.

At first I was worried about confusion as to open or closed magazine flap but found that, reaching back for a magazine, my hand instantly telegraphed flap or open carry. Ideal? Maybe not. But at least I'm not groping for a nonexistent item. It's on my belt and in the same general body area.

Eddie mentioned his losing his magazines from his IPSC-type magazine holders during a high-speed jeep chase across the desert when he was running down rustlers. Eddie learned a lesson from that and now knows that for his work, IPSC magazine holders are poison.

Gun Belt over Clothing

As I said, I've learned to place the filled gun belt over a sweater or sweatshirt, placing it above and directly onto the pants gun belt underneath. This has proven to be a very stable and surprisingly comfortable variation of the two-gun belt system.

Gluing Items onto the Gun Belt

Over the years, I've developed another idea that definitely adds to the security of the items that are kept on the gun belt. (This only works if the gun belt is used as a second over-belt to the pant gun belt.) I simply glue the holsters, magazine pouches, and other item holders to the exact area on the gun belt that conforms to the area I want them. This stops them from shifting around on the belt and allows me to hang said belt on a hook without the filled magazines, etc., shifting around with gravity. Contact cement works wonderfully well for this task as long as the surfaces glued are flat, thus forming a tight seal.

Pocket Magazine Pouches

Another trick I've developed is cutting the flap off a military double-web pouch in .45 ACP and, after filling it with two .45 magazines, sticking it into a back pocket. Another such set-up can be stuck in the other back pocket. This allows many filled magazines to be carried comfortably concealed and protected from all manner of dirt and lint—not to mention how it saves today's thin pockets from being holed. This is excellent if one does not want to use the belt carry for all the ammo or wants even more ammo (it works best with single-column magazines).

Once again, uniformity deems that all magazines be ensconced in the same general area. My hand reaches back for a magazine and instantly tells me pocket or belt area—a compro-

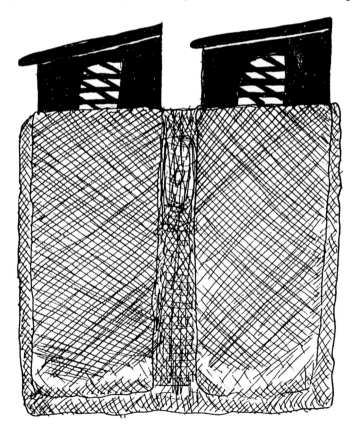

POCKET MAGAZINE POUCH: An old military double-web pouch with flap cut away makes a dandy pocket pouch.

mise to be sure, but again, not a life-threatening one since the general area my hand reaches does contain what I'm looking for.

A belt holster must be comfortable enough to be carried throughout the day. To do this, it is important to balance everything on the belt. Proper balance is critical to comfort and stability. It is much more important than how heavy the items are that the belt supports. When this is done correctly, you will be surprised to discover that two pistols on a belt, properly balanced, are more comfortable than one pistol alone.

The same goes for magazines. Distribute the weight evenly and the weight seems to almost vanish. For one-gun carry, have your magazines on the opposite side for balance.

For street use, it is important that you be able to draw your pistol and extra magazines with ease and with one hand while driving a car, walking, running, climbing, sitting, or prone. The belt holster should be safe and tight-fitting so that some street punk doesn't have an easy time taking your handgun away from you. I prefer a well-fitted holster that has been boned to the pistol in it to one relying on straps for retention. You also want it rugged enough so that it can't be ripped open if someone tries to snatch your pistol from it.

Avoid extra doodads, hidden buttons, swivels, and so on like the plague. Keep it all simple, and you'll find that Murphy's Law has a hard time getting at you.

If you anticipate being in the field, on horseback, or in a bouncing jeep, you may want a duplicate rig that uses retaining straps (with a tight-fitting holster) and magazine flaps on all pouches. For these special purposes, added weapon and accouterment security is needed over extra speed.

STREET SURVIVAL LESSONS

1) *Buy quality.* Cheap accessories and accouterments, like junk guns, are a very poor investment that can lower your odds of street survival.

2) *Test many rigs.* See what rig really works best for you.

I find a variation of one of Hardin's ideas—a brace of handguns carried in the front draw position, waist high, butts forward—suits the bill nicely for me.

3) *A brace of matching handguns and a long gun.* I prefer to wear a brace of handguns even when I carry a long gun, since the long gun may not be in my hands at the moment I need it. The handguns will always be there with enough ammo.

4) *Ammo uniformity for most of us.* Don't complicate life more than it is. Keep the ammo of the same weight and velocity in all your magazines, that is unless you are a SWAT team member or a specialist with special needs.

5) *Use the tactical reload sparingly.* The tactical reload should not be used as a routine, matter-of-course technique, but only for situations where an enemy position is to be stormed.

6) *Double belly band rig.* The use of this rig allows one to carry a matching brace of concealed handguns.

7) *Beware of IPSC magazine holders.* For street use, never use IPSC holders unless you want that extra speed and can afford to lose a magazine or two because you have so many more on you in closed pouches and, hopefully, a backup handgun.

8) *Gluing items to your gun belt.* Gluing holsters, pouches, etc. to your gun belt helps keep everything in place.

High-Ride Holster

It seems that many people spend more time sitting in cars or behind desks than walking. Because of this, they prefer the high-ride type of holster whenever possible. This goes for the relatively few in number that ride horseback.

In the car or at the desk, high-ride hip holsters are best carried in front of the hip rather than over the kidney area. This is because the seat pushes them into one's back.

Ankle Holster

Many experts of holster design consider the ankle holster to be one of the very best of concealment holsters. Today, with the number of cut-down and lightweight semiautos around in major calibers, one does not have to rely solely on Chief or Detective Special snub-nosed revolvers anymore. While many consider this a comfortable holster, I must confess to being in a small group that does not share their enthusiasm. My ankle and leg bones just don't like anything strapped to them, padded or not. I also find ankle holsters quite difficult to wear unless the pant style in vogue is one of those nice times for ankle holsters, such as when bell-bottoms or wide cuffs are in.

The ankle holster is excellent if you are seated at a desk or in a car where your gun hand can reach down for it with ease, since your pant leg is somewhat up your leg. In this position, the one-handed draw can be carried out with ease. It even has its place if you are knocked to the ground in that you still should be able to reach it with one hand.

The problem arises when you are standing. You must pull your pant leg up with both hands, then, still holding the pants up, draw the pistol with your strong hand. Try to do this while Atilla the Hun is breathing down your throat and you will quickly see the error of your ways. Another problem is when walking or running. This is a holster system that necessitates your having to come to a full stop in order to draw your weapon. By golly, if that isn't a drawback, I don't know what is.

Is there a use for the ankle holster? Yes, I believe so. It is ideally suited for a third or fourth handgun where speed may not be as critical a factor. It also can park a hideout gun there, though most street punks are wise to it. Whatever

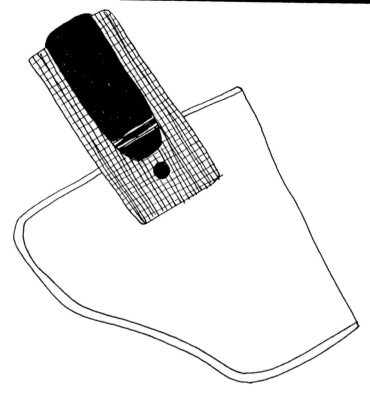

MODIFIED CLIP HOLSTER: I have found that by removing the metal clip from a waistband-type pouch holster and reattaching it higher up the pouch, one can hide a small auto or revolver from view when the clip is put on the waistband or pocket edge. A practical idea waiting a holster maker.

choice you make, be sure you do it uniformly. Use an ankle holster all the time if you like them. This holster can really get you hurt if you are someone who wears a belt holster all day and then decides to switch to an ankle holster at night. If you desperately need a gun, you may find yourself reaching for a belt gun that's not there. Such foolishness could cost you your life.

Crotch Holster
This is an area of the male torso that is usually repugnant to other males and is therefore a very good place to hide a

small hideout handgun. In routine body searches by males, this area of the anatomy is almost always lightly skirted, unless the searchers are forewarned of the possibility of its being a hiding spot or they are real pros.

You must admit the crotch is a novel place to carry a small undercover gun. Of course, it is difficult to speed draw from and could raise eyebrows as you unzip your fly and pull out your weapon.

The crotch holster is secured by a piece of leather that connects to the inside of your belt. I've tried to carry a pistol there but gave up on the idea as being too slow in the draw for a backup gun. A Star PD hides somewhat uncomfortably even if your pants are loose fitting! A pair of tight jeans is definitely not the way to go with a crotch holster. With proper trousers, though, it does make a dandy place for a tiny hideout gun (third or fourth gun) as long as the muzzle of the handgun does not point directly at a vital organ.

Armpit Holster

If you think a shoulder holster smells like death warmed over in hot climates, try an armpit holster. This is only for cold climates and for nothing larger than a .38 snubby. The holster hangs down outside the weak side sleeve secured by a button, the gun butt in a forward position. It can be surprisingly fast when pulled from under a suit coat or jacket. It seems to avoid detection even in a determined frisk, in that it is a very rare holster for daily wear and is passed by. Once again, unless you have a special need for this kind of concealment, leave it for that third or fourth handgun, and, even then, remember that the muzzle of the gun is pointing directly at you.

Wrist Holster

These were once popular when men wore very loose sleeves. It can still be a method of carry if the climate is cold and the handgun is thin and very small. Once again, this is a very specialized setup for a very peculiar concealment problem that goes against the clothing style of the day.

Leg Holster

Leg holsters are usually very uncomfortable, though some improvements have been made in design. Unless you wear a kilt or dress, it is almost impossible to draw your handgun without almost getting undressed. Once again, this is a very peculiar solution to the problem of concealment.

Shoulder Holster: Horizontal Carry

I have never been a fan of shoulder holsters, though devotees of this mode of carry certainly are not lacking.

Living in a climate that can be warm most of the year, I find they tend to get mangy and smelly in short order. When I do carry one, it is always of the vertical-carry design, not one of those horizontal-carry jobs (though wonderful for quick draw) that break a more important rule than that of uniformity—the rule of safety. I never could understand how people could go out in the street with their gun barrel pointing at everyone they just passed. Putting a Glock pistol with its trigger safety system into one of these contraptions is what I would call living dangerously. How easy it would be to squeeze that trigger when grasping the pistol in the stress of combat. You might have a hard time in court explaining why your pistol fired and hit that innocent child walking behind you.

Shoulder Holster: Upside Down

Another shoulder holster variation that leaves me cold is the upside down carry in which the handgun barrel points up at the armpit of its master. Pointing gun muzzles in such a manner, while popular in some quarters, is once again a clear violation of the rules of gun safety and lends itself to tragedy, especially with those Glock pistols, the H&K P7 squeeze cocker design, and, for that matter, any handgun. Think about it. Is it worth it?

Pocket Holster

Carrying a handgun in the pocket is feasible, though much more difficult than in the old days when pockets were pockets and were made to carry serious weights constructed and designed with this task in mind. Some of today's pockets resemble the fake bumpers that appeared on some of the cars of the early 1960s; they look like pockets but don't function like pockets. You put things in them and they easily tear and develop large holes. Or upon even the slightest exertion, they spit out their contents.

Here again, holsterless carry is a mistake. Use a good inside-the-pocket holster manufactured by a good holster maker. You may have to carry small-size handguns, since most serious-caliber handguns are too large for this task. Exceptions do exist if those pockets are large enough. I have found the S&W Bodyguard and Centennial series to be extremely well suited to the task they were designed for. Also, some of the small hammerless or hammer-enclosed automatics work very well. Once again, I'd find this an acceptable idea if carried along with a brace of .45 autos on the belt. I do not like them as primary guns, though many, my daughters included, would disagree.

Holster Fasteners

If you want to use a fastener to hold your handgun in a street holster, don't use one of those retaining strap designs that goes over the trigger guard. Such contraptions can easily be caught between your hand and the gun's trigger guard in the heat of the moment. Also, there have been reports of accidental discharges with revolvers when retaining straps were secured in this position. Better to have the retaining strap pass over the area of the hammer.

Another problem is the use of long retaining straps. Avoid these and go for the shorter types. If I were using a holster with a retaining strap (I've cut all of mine away), I would go for the thumb-snap design. It's efficient and just about foolproof.

"Mexican Carry"

Carrying a handgun in the waistband is a popular method of carry for those who have no time or use for holsters. Sticking a handgun into your belt "Mexican" is a sure formula for doom since the impact of collision between you and

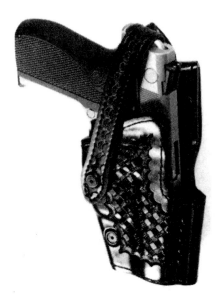

SAFARILAND HOLSTER WITH RETAINING STRAP: The correct length strap is placed over the hammer, not over the trigger guard.

some attacking street nut almost certainly will send it crashing to the ground and out of reach, or worse, into his hands. I admit to having been guilty in the past of using such a carry. I found that the handgun had a tendency to slowly shift around and came to the conclusion that the Mexican carry was not only an unstable way to carry a handgun needed for close-quarter life-saving chores, but actually extremely unsafe in many aspects. For instance, Glock pistols can have their triggers squeezed inadvertently by clothing, cocked and locked single-action semiautos can have their slide safeties pushed down, and so on.

When in uniform and out in the field, I grew to respect those U.S. Ordnance officers at the turn of the century who pushed for a grip safety to be placed on the Colt 1911. Once or twice I looked down at my customized Colt 1911 after some strenuous exercise to find that the extended slide safety had been pushed out of position. U.S. Army Ordnance knew what they were doing when they insisted on standard 1911 slide safeties for military use. It would be prudent to keep this in mind when using a handgun in the field. Looking down at the slide safety in the fire position reminded me that the grip safety on the 1911 is definitely not an affectation but a useful safety feature.

Another drawback of the holsterless belt carry is having the handgun fall from place and into the pants. More than once I had to extract a small Star PD from my pant leg. I came to the conclusion that this was a very ridiculous situation that drastically cut down my chances for street survival. I now have dropped any notion of using holsterless belt carry.

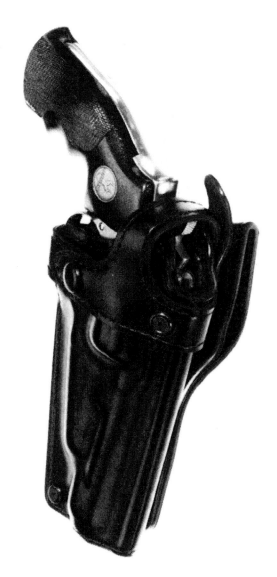

SAFARILAND HOLSTER WITH THUMB BREAK: I don't much like holster fasteners except for military use, but if I kept them on my holsters, I would prefer the thumb-break design.

Taped-to-the-Body Hideout Gun

Taping a tiny handgun to the body is a popular way for some to hide an emergency hideout gun. The small of the back is a very popular area for such a gun in that it may go unnoticed in a body search. Even if the area is "wiped" by the hands, if the tape is smooth and clothing is worn, the searcher may miss it.

Another favorite spot is the inside of the upper arm, for the same reason. Such tactics have their place, and everyone, especially officers of the law, should be aware of this.

Case Study: Don't Go Off Half-Cocked

I have a good friend named Nate. Nate is sort of an urban cowboy, enamored to wearing 10-gallon hats, string ties, and cowboy boots. All this in Jerusalem. A few years back he paid me a visit and, after a time, asked me one of his endless questions pertaining to guns. He's what we could affectionately call a "gun nut." One day, Nate pulled his Colt .45 Combat Commander and asked me if it was safe to carry it on half-cock safety. I assured him it was not, and that this so-called "safety," if I correctly recalled from an article in the *American Rifleman* magazine years ago, was there only to catch the hammer if it slipped forward by accident when the slide was pulled back.

Now this just didn't satisfy Nate, who went on to question the quality of my memory. I repeated the contention that making his extremely safe Colt unsafe was the height of stupidity and that he would regret this foolish act. After we watched a good Western on my VCR, he bid me adieu. I felt that I had somehow not impressed upon him the error of his ways.

It wasn't a month later when there was a knock on my door. Looking through an opaque glass window, I saw his 10-gallon hat shadowed against the sunlight. When I opened the door, he was standing there wide-eyed, as he pulled a pair of jockey shorts from a paper bag. They looked like they had been rescued from a fire in the nick of time. On top of this, the seat of the shorts had sustained some sort of an explosion. It was blown away, hanging, torn to shreds.

He sputtered out the story. Seems he was at the airport servicing a candy store that he owned and had taken his half-cocked Combat Commander and stuck it into his belt Mexican carry, right over the right kidney. Opening his car's rear trunk, he bent over to lift a load of candy out when he heard a loud explosion and felt the rear of his pants. They were on fire.

He jumped around trying to put out the flames and finally succeeded, losing a pair of slacks and jockey shorts in the bargain. He felt it was mighty lucky no one else was around. Holding the shorts out, he said he shuddered to think what would have transpired if he put the pistol behind his belt buckle. Obviously, his clothing had somehow pulled that hammer over the half-cock notch. One helluva close call . . .

STREET SURVIVAL LESSONS

1) *Use a holster.* Never carry a handgun Mexican carry; you almost certainly will lose it in a hassle.

2) *Be aware of taped hideout guns.* Securing tiny handguns by tape to the skin can be a very easy technique of carrying and hiding them. Some criminals have even taken to hiding such weapons in their intestinal tract by insertion into the anus.

3) *Know holster fasteners.* Know the do's and don'ts of the use of holster fasteners. Poorly designed ones can get you hurt.

4) *Don't go off half-cocked.* Never carry a Colt 1911 or any clone on half-cock safety unless you're contemplating suicide.

TILTING THE ODDS IN YOUR FAVOR

The battle against the street predator is an unfair one. The street predator can choose the time, the place, and his victim. He does not obey the law and is therefore not restricted in the type or use of the weapon he carries. We are.

While we are entangled in a maze of laws that almost seem written to cut down our chances of survival, the street predator is immune to all that. Many times we cannot even carry our defensive weaponry in a manner that gives us even a fighting chance in a close-quarter surprise ambush. We are playing on an uneven playing field.

While governments around the globe frame laws that seemingly cut down our chances of coping with brutal attack, we must grope for answers that will tilt back the negative odds we face. The situation can be quite confusing, as there is no uniform way to do this since the laws and social-acceptance standards of each nation can differ quite dramatically. For example, in some nations the display of edged weapons is legal and socially acceptable. In others. such a display can get you arrested in short order. In some nations, carrying rifles and submachine guns is deemed normal while cocked and locked pistols will raise eyebrows or worse. All this has an important effect on how we dress for the street, yet how we cope with this problem does have a very practical and direct effect on our survival.

Close-Quarter Knife Attack: Will You Be Bloodied?

Top experts say you cannot draw your handgun and defend yourself against a trained knife wielder who rushes at you from 8 yards. He can cover the distance in about 1.5 seconds. They claim that, regardless of your skills, you must be prepared to be sliced and stabbed in your weak hand as you draw your handgun with your strong hand. Is this true? From what I have seen in the streets of Israel, where such attacks are commonplace, the answer is a resounding yes. You will almost certainly be bloodied unless you already have your weapon in hand.

Facing this reality, I set about trying to solve the seemingly impossible problem of having a handgun in hand while appearing unarmed. It became obvious that walking around with gun in hand would not only get me arrested, but, in the tense atmosphere, might even get me shot by the first police officer or soldier who spotted me, not to mention the armed citizenry. Could a satisfactory answer be found? After much research and testing, I believe it has.

Looking Unarmed while Armed to the Teeth

Finding a technique that allows one to walk with handgun in hand while no one spots it is a very difficult problem, one that almost defies solution. The need to accomplish this in a manner that allows one to be comfortable for long periods of time and still allows one to engage an enemy or enemies in a 360-degree traverse of fire in an instant certainly adds to the problem.

In time, I came to the conclusion that the ultimate solution that had eluded so many was almost in the realm of the surreal. Each and every expert I consulted told me it could not be done. I was cautioned that one had to accept the fact that an attacker would draw blood unless the gun was already in hand, and that having a gun in hand in the manner I stipulated was quite impossible. I could not accept this thesis. I felt there had to be a way.

The Cane Defense

I set about learning how to use a cane as an extension of my weak hand in a manner that would ward off an attacker while I drew my handgun. The cane defense is probably the best of the many ideas that can be used to do this in that it acts as a buffer between you and your attacker—a buffer that has no vital nerves or blood vessels. Unfortunately, unless the cane has a razor-sharp edge and point (then it's a sword), it really does not win you too much time, since it is wielded by the weak hand in a relatively inefficient manner. Using it in the more effective strong hand means that you would not be able to draw the handgun as efficiently as warranted. It was a toss-up. I therefore went for the weak-hand cane carry, since getting at that handgun as fast as possible was still the first priority.

The Armored Glove

The idea of the armored glove has reappeared after centuries of lying dormant. The knights of old used armored gloves to ward off the blows of bladed weapons. Such gloves increase your chances of not getting cut, allowing you to really grapple with an attacker as you use the strong hand to draw your handgun. This piece of equipment has its merits and may prove useful to the uniformed officer who cannot work with drawn weapon in hand.

Hand in the Fanny Pack or Purse

Since I prefer the technique of handgun in the hand, I kept on experimenting with methods that allowed me to do this.

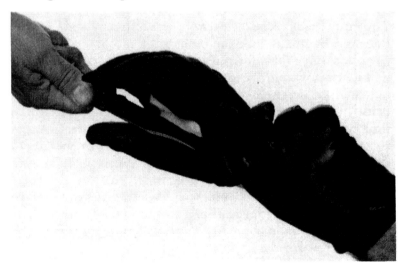

HATCH "RESISTER GLOVE": A quality product that offers greater hand protection against blade cuts and needle punctures, the Kevlar knit liner and leather glove #RFK 300 are still thin enough for practical use out in the street.

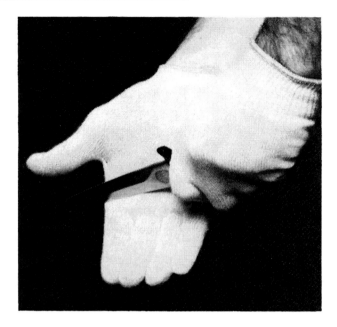

HATCH KEVLAR KNIT LINER.

The fanny pack or purse carry opened up a new approach. Putting a hand into an open fanny pack or purse allows one to at least have the handgun somewhat ready for instant use and is comfortable for long periods of time when properly adjusted for height. The big problem was that I still had to draw the weapon, a task that took time and forced me to limit my traverse of fire in the first crucial seconds. Enemies to my rear or side still took longer to engage than enemies to the front. While this may seem like hair splitting, I was convinced that each increment of time between me and success was something to be eliminated. I wanted those negative odds to swing in my favor. While a hand in the fanny pack or purse was an improvement, it still wasn't the answer. The odds still favored the street predator.

The Napoleon Carry
In working with Israelis faced with walking narrow streets filled with potential killers, I suggested what I call the Napoleon carry. In this technique, the handgun is drawn and

placed under the cover of one's open jacket or vest, much as the hand of the emperor Napoleon appears in his many portraits. (Historians claim Napoleon suffered from some affliction whose pain was partially alleviated by the warmth of his hand.) The problem with this carry is the discomfort that ensues with holding the hand in such a fashion for very long periods of time.

I still had to contend with the speed of the draw. Engaging front and back targets was still too slow for my taste. I wanted another answer, one that approached the ideal of walking with my gun in hand, ready for instant reaction to a close-quarter ambush. It was clear to me that, while useful, this method of carry still did not fill the bill.

The Pocketless Carry

A novel way of carrying that I came up with was the actual elimination of the pocket of a jacket or coat. The hand stayed in the pocket slit, but the pocket was actually removed. I found the system worked fine for direct attacks but still gave me restricted traverse capability to engage attacks from the side and the rear. It still didn't satisfy me.

The Newspaper Carry

Spending months in the street testing different techniques of having handgun in hand while still appearing unarmed had taken me through the full gauntlet of possibilities. I knew that Chicago gangsters had carried handguns concealed by newspapers, so I tested the idea. In time I became convinced that if such a technique had been used, it most probably had not been used for long-term carry but rather to carry out assassinations, the gun being covered only when it was about to be used. I found the technique looked quite artificial and strange. People do not walk down the street with their hands and forearms covered by the *Evening News*.

The Arm in the Sling Carry

Having your arm in a sling does allow for a small pistol to be carried in a covert way. Reaction speed is quite good if you learn the trick of using a weak breakaway thread to hold the sling around your neck. In time I realized that this worked best for small handguns only and that the angle of carry was just too awkward. Another problem was the fact that the sling tended to be conspicuous. Walking around that way (same for the cane) elicited endless questions about "how did that happen?" I soon dropped this idea along with all the rest except for the Napoleon carry, growing more and more frustrated as I accepted the possibility that there was indeed no practical answer to the problem. Then it happened . . .

Solution: The Grab-Bag Carry
I had a fleeting memory of something I had read years before. A handgun had been carried in a paper bag and had been used that way in a killing. Could this be the long-awaited answer to the problem? I rushed downstairs, opened a broom closet, and searched for paper bags. There were not any to be had. What I did have was a plastic tote bag that had finger slots. I rushed upstairs and took a Colt 1911 in hand. It was well concealed. Of course, there also was the problem of proper functioning to contend with. The use of a semiauto, while theoretically feasible, still needed to be tested.

My eyes wandered to the wall, where a S&W 1917 in .45 ACP hung. Taking it down, I placed my fingers into one of

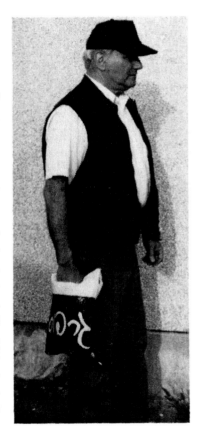

THE GRAB-BAG CARRY. An excellent method of carrying a concealed handgun in the hand ready for instant use.

the slots, put the revolver in my hand, and then put my thumb through the other slot.

It worked. The long sought-after answer to the puzzle was at hand. A handgun in a plastic bag fitted with finger slots was highly concealable, yet allowed for the gun to be point-fired at a close-quarter attacker.

I soon realized that the bag I had chosen was much too large in that it flapped around when the handgun was raised and pointed, I spotted another bag that was smaller and the problem ceased. More testing showed that even an 8 3/8-inch-barreled S&W frame could be carried in a bag 10 inches by 14.5 inches. As I tested many handguns by point shooting, it soon became evident that the system worked. Now here was an idea with enormous possibilities. I named the new system the "grab bag." The following became evident:

a) The system works if one is careful not to catch the hammer.

If one is neat and careful this will not occur. A striker-fired semiauto like the Glock or a "hammerless" revolver worked best. (I am currently experimenting with a strip of cardboard glued to the top of the bag that prevents hammers from catching.)

b) The longer the barrel, the more stable the bag, supported through it's full length.

c) The finger-slotted bag allowed a very firm grip to be taken, far superior to what, say, a plain paper bag would allow.

d) Here was another drawback: you had to use a dark bag or light might shine through and highlight the handgun.

e) The grab bag is comfortable for long periods of carry in that the bag can be held down at the side and looks natural.

f) It allows a full 360-degree traverse of fire, which picks up multiple close-quarter targets with ease using point fire.

g) Point shooting is a natural system for the grab bag, working best in hip-fire but also in quick-fire if needed.

h) The bag acts as a carrier for the handgun when you are seated in someone's home or at work, etc. Placing the grab

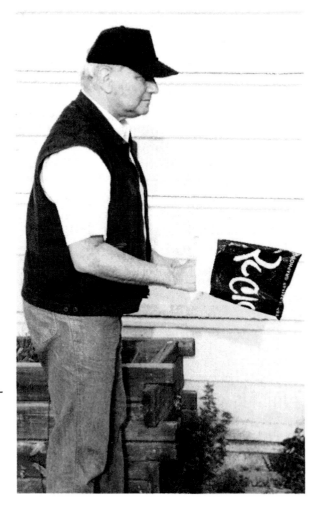

POINT—HIP FIRE WITH THE GRAB BAG: The grab-bag system is ideal for close-quarter instinctive fire.

bag on my lap raises no eyebrows or unwanted questions. Anyone checking the bag deems it acceptable that the hand-gun is being transported this way.

STREET SURVIVAL LESSON

1) *The grab bag.* There is now a practical, low-cost solution to having a concealed gun in the hand

that works for long periods of carry time and allows 360-degree traverse of fire if you are faced with a charging, knife-wielding adversary.

BODY ARMOR

The last decade or two has shown very marked improvements in low-cost, lightweight, soft body armor. Now, for the first time since the common man first fashioned body armor out of leather and wood (knights of old had them made out of iron), body armor is available to all and sundry.

The problem with body armor is that it still is the bane of those wearing it in hot climates. Heat, not weight, is a problem that remains to be solved and is the reason most individuals except street cops, SWAT team members, and those in the military avoid them like the plague and don't wear them with any degree of regularity.

With improvements in design, the problem of tell-tale signs that you're wearing one is almost nonexistent except to the trained eye on the lookout for such things.

Is body armor needed for street survival? In my opinion, most decidedly, yes. It is as necessary as the weapon you carry, but I venture to guess only one civilian in 10,000 will wear it day in and day out—the heat problem, you see.

Here in Israel, terrorists have learned that most uniformed police and soldiers wear some sort of body armor and so have devised their attacks, especially with bladed weapons, to target the throat and neck of their victims. Because of this, we see an inordinate amount of victims being wheeled to ambulances with knives sticking into this area of the anatomy. (Never pull a knife out until at a hospital, or the victim may bleed to death. The knife acts as a stopper.)

I wear soft body armor when I know I will walk in the crowded open-air marketplace. Rubbing shoulders and elbows with potential terrorists makes me forget the heat problem. Another time is when I drive in areas highly prone to ambush. It's a compromise, one that I and others could regret, but this book is written to help you the reader and not to impress you with this writer's alleged infallibility. So in the interest of candor, I caution that in this case, do as I say and not as I do. Most certainly, police officers and the military, when in a combat situation, should wear their body armor at all times.

For civilians who want to know when to compromise on wearing it, I can only recommend that you try to pick the occasions that you feel you may most need it, keeping in mind that this is only a very semieducated guesstimate that you, too, could regret to your dying day.

Armor against Knives

Body armor is usually thought of as being a defense against bullets and is graded as to its ability to defeat various velocity, caliber, and weight combinations. When we come up against knives, we face a problem. With knives, the smaller the caliber the more effective they can be in penetrating soft body armor. An ice pick is a super penetrator and will defeat most types of soft body armor. In many ways, ice picks resemble armor-piercing ammo. The same is true for stilettos, thin daggers, and triangular-bladed OSS daggers of the type used during World War II. Wider, larger knives, especially those with blunter tips, tend to have a more difficult time defeating Kevlar vests, though they can do it.

Ceramic inserts meant to stop rifle bullets will do the trick, but they and metallic inserts are usually too heavy and unwieldy for daily use. I can remember visiting a police supply store in New England, where I had gone to purchase a soft body armor vest. Engaging in conversation with the proprietor, he told me a story about a salesman who had tried to sell him his brand of soft body armor. He said the salesman sat down, placed the body armor on his thigh, and while loudly lauding its alleged knife-defeating capabilities, grabbed a dagger from the display case and plunged it into the vest. As the two ambulance attendants wheeled him out of the store, he still insisted knives can't defeat soft body armor. Seems myths die hard deaths.

Soft body armor tends to be at its best against knife slashes rather than stabs. It acts like the leather jackets so favored by street gangs when they engage in knife fights. These jackets are fairly dependable in protecting one from slashers, but not from stabbers who use strong, sharp-pointed, thin-bladed knives.

I have seen a new type of body armor made in Israel that resembles chain mail but is made of some kind of metal, possibly hardened aluminum or titanium. It is very lightweight and has the ability to breathe, making it suited for warm weather. I believe it will defeat knife slash attacks, and though it just might stop most knife stabs, ice picks would still be a very big problem. It is still being tested.

As I was writing, this bit of information came across my desk that may be the big breakthrough in stab-proof armor we have all been waiting for. First Chance Armor and Equipment of Brockton, Massachusetts, has just announced the development of a new material and process that produces a soft, flexible, stab-resistant vest that defeats bullets and knives, including ice picks. If so, it has made a tremendous advance in protective armor, one of major significance and importance to street survival.

BARREL COMPENSATORS OUT ON THE STREET

More and more handguns sporting built-in barrel compensators are appearing on guns for competition. Being ever lighter in weight and more compact, some are now being carried out in the street. Whether this is an improvement or not is a moot question. If someone feels that a particular thing helps him shoot better, it can act (as long as it is not detrimental) as a big booster to self-confidence. The idea of carrying one's competition gun and rig in the street certainly coexists with the principle of uniformity. Carrying what you practice with is, of course, the way to go. Some street-worthy comp guns are even the same weight and size as the standard-model handgun. Great strides have been made since they first appeared as competition-only guns.

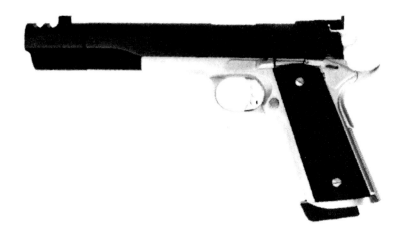

COLT CUSTOM COMP: A compensated Colt for sport that some like for street carry. While this is possible, most would find this particular slide length a little excessive.

One thing to look out for in carrying a barrel-compensated gun in the street is the potential problem of powder flash. Almost all competition shooting is done in daylight, and some shooters never fire their handguns in low light or dark conditions. This goes for some police and military training programs as well. I make it a point to do lots of shooting in nondaylight hours.

It is amazing how many problems arise, and one of them could be the temporary blinding of the shooter by muzzle flash, especially muzzle flash created by burning gasses flaming above and in front of one's hybrid compensated street gun. This is especially true when one uses a high-pressure caliber as the hot 10mm. High-pressure calibers such as the 10mm benefit the most from barrel compensators. But if you are going to carry such a weapon, make sure you test-fire the compensator at night. I hope you aren't unpleasantly surprised to find that the latest hot set-up design of compensator on your handgun doesn't hurt your night vision as all those hot gasses explode in a sheet of bright flame. This may not happen, but check it out. You don't want to find yourself temporarily blinded in a close-quarter confrontation.

Some of the newer designs have reportedly cut down muzzle flash and would be a welcome change if, in fact, they do as advertised. Incidentally, military ammo usually exhibits less muzzle flash than most brands of commercial ammo.

It's important to do most of your practice shooting under poor light conditions. After all, street predators prefer the cloak of darkness to carry out their nefarious deeds.

Some may worry about the loss of velocity when using barrel compensators, but this has not proven to be a very justifiable fear. Velocity loss is slight but consistent—certainly not enough to cut down stopping power, though I would check your street-carry ammo in a good chronograph just to be extra sure.

One thing a compensated handgun does do is increase the practical accuracy of the shooter. Group sizes are cut, some by as much as half, because felt recoil, muzzle jump, and recovery time are all reduced, helping to keep those sights on target.

Theoretically, this should increase hit probability as well as smoothing out the acquisition of multiple targets. Whether you use your sights or the more practical point-shooting method at close range, this should be a plus. But I caution you to try out your friend's competition comp at night before you butcher up that barrel and slide.

LANYARDS ON PISTOLS

At one time, the use of lanyards on handguns was considered as normal as riding a horse for transportation. One had only to have his handgun fall from his hand and be lost in the sagebrush to become a true believer in the practicality of lanyards. Alas, we travel by vehicle today, and the lanyard has been deemed an obsolete affectation on modern handguns. But is it? Is there still a practical use for lanyards, other than for people on horseback? The answer, according to Jonathan, is a very resounding yes.

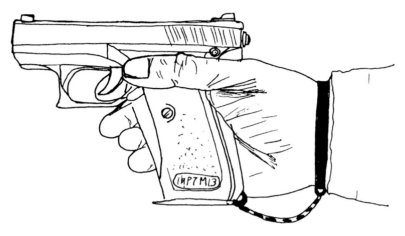

WRIST LANYARD.

E.S.: Where in heaven's name do you see the use of lanyards in this day and age except for those on horseback?

J: In special operations, where the handgun is your primary weapon, I developed the use of a short wrist lanyard in my SWAT team days, using them to secure the handgun to my wrist when we kicked down a door. The trick was to use a lanyard that was only of enough length to secure the handgun to a leather bracelet on the wrist. The traditional lanyard gets in the way, and I found it unsuited for this work. The short lanyard, being only a few inches in length, works quite well in that you can't trip over it or get tangled up. If the handgun falls from your grasp, it is still within easy reach to be grasped once again. I have pushed the concept for special unit work.

E.S.: So this is not theoretical?

J: No, sir. It's been used in many SWAT operations with quite satisfactory results.

....

STREET SURVIVAL LESSONS

1)   *Soft body armor against knives.* The use of body armor for the police and military is a must. What

must not be forgotten is its use for the average civilian who has charted the areas where drive-by shootings have occurred or for those living in countries where close-quarter attacks are a daily occurrence. Standard soft body armor can sometimes be defeated by slashing knifes. It does poorly against stabbing attacks and is easily defeated by ice picks. The new millennium vest may change all this.

2) *Barrel compensators work in the street.* In theory, and after testing, barrel compensators can help in street survival if one shoots better with them. The same goes for all competition-type equipment if it does not interfere with proper weapon use and helps tilt the odds in your favor.

3) *Lanyards are not obsolete for special purposes.* The use of the lanyard, modified for SWAT use in its short configuration and unmodified in length for horseback, is still valid.

Chapter Six

The Street

*E*ven in the crime-ridden atmosphere of the end of the twentieth century, there are still areas deemed bad neighborhoods and bad parts of town. There are also bad locales, such as sleazy drinking clubs. I remember reading a question once that asked, "How can I avoid fights in biker bars?" The answer was a gem of country wisdom: "Don't go to them."

AREA AVOIDANCE: THE BEST POLICY?

Avoidance is a policy that has its merits. The problem is, it's becoming more and more impossible to avoid the danger in our streets as mindless violence spreads like a cancerous amoeba across the globe. Living by the policy of avoidance grossly restricts our personal freedom and is an assault on our right to pursue happiness. While it may have worked only a decade ago, it now is becoming an increasingly academic activity. Even at home, locked behind the best security systems money can buy, the street oozes between the cracks and holes in our supposedly airtight defense like something out of a B science fiction flick.

Avoidance is a dying tactic. The street just won't go away. It's time to face the challenge and conquer it.

THE INSTANT RECONNOITER

Whenever you leave the confines of your home or vehicle, enter a room, or are about to turn the corner of a street, it would behoove you to cultivate a tactic I call the instant reconnoiter. Learn the trick of moving those wonderful orbs in your head called eyes across the panorama of the area you are about to enter. Are there any telltale dangers out there, such as dark shadows, poor lighting, obstacles where some street predator could wait in ambush? Do you notice a suspicious character standing in the shadows? A group of young men milling about under some street lamp? A car moving slowly down the street? Learn to instantly take in a photographic picture of the new environment you are about to enter. Like the good Colonel Baum, have an instant picture of the "battlefield" burned into your mind.

In studying cases of terrorist attacks on hapless victims going about their daily tasks and duties, I've found one upsetting ingredient repeated itself over and over. They were simply blindly unaware of the danger they were moving into. They looked but they did not receive. It was as if they were nonchalantly walking to an easy chair in their living room rather than encroaching on an obviously suspicious character waiting with a butcher knife in a bag. Sometimes only blind luck saved their lives.

Case Study: Bus Stop Attack at Neveh Yaakov

Neveh Yaakov is a small suburb of north Jerusalem that has seen more than its share of terror attacks. It was against this backdrop that a young Israeli soldier came to a bus stop in the wee hours of one of those wonderful Jerusalem mornings. Road traffic was light except for a few produce-laden trucks making for market. The soldier stood there on the lonely, deserted sidewalk, oblivious to his environment, not sweeping the area with his eyes. Suddenly, the early morning tranquillity was broken by a blood-curdling cry behind him of *"Allah Akhbar!"* He turned to see a huge knife raised above his head. Fortunately, our young soldier was in peak physical condition and had reflexes to match. They say that's what saved his life as he grappled with his male Arab attacker, getting cut up in the process.

Now our young soldier had a problem. His M16 was unloaded and didn't even have a magazine in it. So while wrestling with the terrorist he had to place the magazine into his M16 and rack a round into its chamber. Believe it or not, he actually succeeded in doing just that. He then preceded to further shatter the peace and quiet with the rip-roaring sound of a full 30-round magazine of 5.56mm military ball ammo, ventilating said perpetrator in a most decisive and final manner. Our soldier, though bloodied, lived to tell the tale.

STREET SURVIVAL LESSONS

1) *Don't daydream.* In the street, don't be oblivious to what's around you. Our young soldier was standing alone in the street, totally oblivious to the remote possibility of danger.

2) *Instant reconnoiter.* Make the instant reconnoiter a natural tool of street survival.

3) *Repeat the reconnoiter.* Act like a radar antenna. Make a sweep of the area as a matter of course. Our young soldier was sleeping with his eyes open.

4) *Never rely on luck for survival.* The excellent physical condition of the soldier saved his life, but this occurred only because the perpetrator verbally signaled his presence with the shout of *"Allah Akhbar!"* This time luck was with the victim; otherwise we would have had one very dead soldier and a terrorist newly armed with an M16 rifle.

5) *Condition #4 is not for the street.* Never go in condition #4. Have a loaded weapon. Added to all the basic errors our young soldier made was the fact that his unloaded rifle made his survival enter the realm of a minor miracle. His ability to load and charge his rifle under such a close-quarter attack was a marvel of manual dexterity, but quite unnecessary if the rifle had been loaded as it should have been. This was not, however, the soldier's fault. The M16 was unloaded because he was obeying standing orders. A bureaucrat had signed a piece of bureaucratic paper deeming the area "safe." Here in the Promised Land, we also have our share of idiots sitting behind desks producing mindless orders and laws that reduce our chances of street survival.

6) *Survival isn't a sin.* Don't be guilty about being alive. The bureaucrats had so confused the issue of street survival that when the young soldier, swathed in bandages, gave a TV interview from his hospital bed, he shyly apologized for shooting his knife-wielding attacker so many times, claiming he wasn't thinking straight. There are those who would beg to differ. When he pumped his attacker full of bullets was the one time the young soldier was thinking straight.

....

No Friends, Only Enemies

During the 1973 Yom Kippur War, a friend who completed his job as chief security officer of the Israeli president's house asked me to work in the narrow streets of the old city section of Jerusalem as a volunteer to the Israeli Police. Kurt was a former Rhodesian who saw service with the British Red Devil paratroopers in the Gulf Emirates. He seemed to have almost a sixth sense in smelling danger.

King wanted me to act as his bodyguard while he went

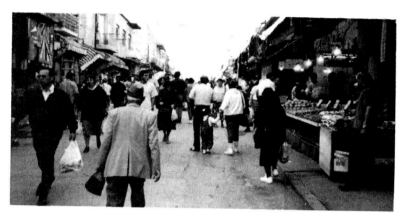

JERUSALEM'S MAHENE YEHUDA SHUK: An open-air marketplace that has been the scene of many terrorist attacks.

about his duties. It was a learning experience par excellence, since I had on-the-job training with the best. We were soon joined by Ami, an undercover agent who wanted to see some action after he was sidelighted by a minor injury. The bonus was he spoke quite excellent Arabic.

During those weeks of around-the-clock patrols in the dark oriental alleys and streets of the open marketplace (*shuk*), one rule was constantly pounded into my head: there are no friends out there in the street, only enemies. If you allow yourself to believe otherwise, you risk leaving this veil of tears called life.

We were sitting outside a small police station called the Kishle on my first night out, covering a group of suspects we had just arrested, when King confided the reason he wanted me with him. True, we were buddies in the same shooting group (the one that Hanon belonged to), and he did feel I would be a good "extra gun" to have along. But there was a second reason. He motioned toward an Arab cop who was sitting behind a desk facing the open front door of the Kishle, transistor radio glued to his ear.

"Smile at him while I talk," he said. I did so, but the sergeant only glared at me. King grinned. "He thinks you're CIA, sent here to help us win the war. That transistor is tuned into Jordan Radio. He's listening to see if King Hussein enters the war. If he does, he has to prove he wasn't a collaborator for us. I'd say he's picked you out as his sacrificial lamb."

Now this threw me for the proverbial loop. "But he's in the Israeli police . . ."

King grinned again. "Him along with just about every other cop at this station. Problem is they're all followers of the prophet Mohammed and will probably do the same as he does or will attempt to do—kill all the Israelis here at the station to prove they're loyal to their cause."

I stared at that transistor radio, then at the murderous look in the sergeant's eye. "King, how many Israelis are here? King played with the swagger stick he kept under his arm, a token of his Red Devil paratroop days. '"Full time? You, me, Ami, maybe another one or two. That's another reason why I wanted you here with me: to cover my ass. Imagine being out on patrol with the likes of that sergeant behind me. Gives me the creeps. Remember, always be suspicious and plan worst-case scenarios for survival. Best-case idealistic ones can get your ass in a sling."

"But why don't you arrest him," I asked.

"Oh, we did arrest two or three who crossed the line and told us what they thought, but you see for political purposes the powers that be have deemed that we continue the fiction that they are loyal police officers."

"That's crazy," I said. King grinned as he tapped some dirt off his boot with the swagger stick. "No, that's politics."

My last night at the Kishle was when the cease-fire was about to be signed. I remember a celebration dinner we were having in an upstairs room. King, Ami, myself, a senior officer, and a Border Police commander were just finishing supper when the radio announced a cease-fire had been signed. The senior officer looked at me and smiled. "America [he called me that], you've had a good experience here. I think you've learned a lot. However, there is one last lesson, one you should never forget if you want to survive. The lesson is, don't be naive. Remember, out there in the street you had no friends. Only King and Ami. Everyone else was a potential enemy. In a few moments there is going to be a knock at that door. Remember that knock when you feel trusting about your fellow human beings."

We made a toast to the cease-fire when the atmosphere was interrupted by a sharp knocking at the door. The senior poked at me and then called out, "Enter." The door swung open and a tray stacked high with cakes and coffee entered the room. Behind it, the sergeant minus the transistor radio beamed, "We won!" He then proceeded to pass out the goodies, smiling at me like his long-lost buddy. Obviously, King Hussein hadn't entered the war.

To this day transistor radios remind me of those days at the Kishle, patrolling the streets and pitch black alleys, the chanting from the tall minarets calling the faithful to prayer, and that sergeant sitting at his desk, staring at me with hatred, transistor radio pressed to his ear.

AMBUSH AVOIDANCE

The very best way of getting the jump on your enemy is through the element of surprise. In classical warfare as well as the warfare of the street, surprise may assume the form of a well-planned ambush. Avoiding ambushes is the best way to ensure that you and your family survive out there in the urban jungle. The trick is how to do it. Is there a plan that can help you avoid ambushes? The answer is a firm yes.

Spotting Crime Patterns

Copycat crimes are almost a staple of the criminal world. Most criminals are not the masterminds that we see in many Hollywood films. Most criminals come from the dregs of society. They are not known for their superabundance of gray matter.

Many will copy what they see as a winning trend, trying to capitalize on it in a most uninventive manner. We have only to read about the latest criminal fad to know how to avoid it. For instance, if I were a tourist in Miami, I certainly would not advertise the fact. Driving in a rental car advertis-

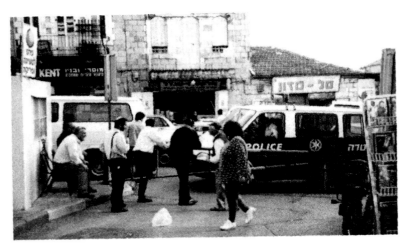

ISRAELI POLICE VAN IN THE SHUK: Since the police can't be everywhere, the ultimate formula for street survival remains within the individual.

es the possibility of your being an out-of-towner. Driving that car into areas of town that the city chamber of commerce deems safe (contrary to crime patterns) proves that you are. Never believe what those city public relations people spout. Read the newspapers, talk to the people on the street. Take cabs. Cab drivers are out there around the clock. They know where the areas of ambush are. They are not infallible. But the mere fact that most survive in the urban jungle speaks wonders for their common sense and street savvy. I would believe their opinions much more than any tourist handbill I read. The cabbie knows his city better than just about anyone. If he didn't, he couldn't ply his trade.

Use a War Map

Get a good street map of the area you intend to travel in. Learn how to read a map so that it is not just a blur of colored lines and symbols. If I lived in a city noted for muggings, attacks on tourists, drive-by shootings, and all the other forms of predator attacks so prevalent today, I would mark each such attack with a specific color on the map. Make a game of it.

Chances are you will see a very distinct pattern emerge for each type of crime. Know where those copycat crime-pattern areas are. Knowledge is intelligence in the military definition. Knowing which areas criminals have been favoring recently can be a big help in street survival.

CRIMINAL TRICKS AND TACTICS

Criminals tend to copy what works. When the local newspapers and TV stations show the latest victim of a crime, criminals watch for helpful clues on what works in the street. What works is a constant topic of conversation among such types. It is no exaggeration to say that most jails and prisons today are schools of crime. Common criminals and terrorists in Israel use such institutions for teaching and indoctrination of their fellow prisoners. They learn all aspects of their evil profession right there at the expense of the state, since it is impossible for any nation to have each and every criminal in solitary confinement. Financial cost and human rights groups would prohibit the practice. Because of this, prisons will continue to be institutions of criminal higher learning.

While you're not in jail with them, you still can be privy to the information they discuss simply by learning to observe and think rather than see. Look at the news media with a trained eye that observes the tricks criminals use. What you see, they see and discuss. Patterns of criminal behavior will emerge, patterns which you must vow never to fall victim to.

Case Study: Ambush in Judea
A favorite trick of Arabs during the beginning of the so-called Intifada was to turn road signs in the wrong direction so that hapless Israeli drivers or hikers would stray from a well-traveled road and wander off into the back country. Many times they went into a well-planned ambush.

One day, our friend Henry had this done to him. Henry is an avid hiker. He hikes all over the country—a true lover of nature who refuses to let anyone tell him that any place is off-limits. He had decided to visit some Israeli settlements about 20 miles south of Jerusalem in an area of hill country that is remote and isolated except for a few less-than-friendly Arab villages. Henry knew that the area was now deemed a "problem area." Cars were being stoned and roadblocks set up to ambush cars on a daily basis. However, Henry reasoned that as long as he hiked in sight of the main road he would be all right. After all, it was still daylight. The army was out patrolling the area. What could go wrong?

Hiking over increasingly rough terrain, Henry looked for the road sign to the Israeli settlement. He smiled as he spotted it and moved off in the direction it pointed. He came upon an unpaved road. About 30 yards from it he noticed two male Arab teenagers staring at him. He waved at them. They didn't wave back. Instead, they grinned malevolently.

As our trusting soul hiked on, he had a gnawing feeling that it was taking him much too long to get to the settlement.

The narrow dirt road seemed to drag on and on. As he came around a bend, he was greeted by a seemingly deserted Arab village; not a soul was in sight. Now this made him somewhat uneasy, but then again, there was that sign. He remembered that sign, so he continued on, but now he left the road and walked through the open fields.

Then all hell broke loose. Curses and loud screams filled the air as the village sprang to life. A mob came out onto the street, onto rooftops. They charged at him, yelling, cursing. A deluge of rocks crashed around him. He took cover behind some rocks, jacked back the slide of his Uzi, and fired a long burst into the air. This seemed to act as a momentary damper on the mob, who melted back into their homes. For the next hour it was like that. A game of cat and mouse as the mob attacked and then was scared back by a burst from Henry's Uzi.

During one attack, the mob suddenly stopped, then ran away in utter silence. Henry turned to see an Israeli Border Police jeep brake and two border policemen armed with M16s jumped out. They made for him. Henry looked down at his Uzi and pulled its magazine. It was almost empty. Henry had gone through six 25-round magazines and was just about to finish the last one when the jeep arrived. He breathed a sigh of relief as the border policemen offered to escort him out of the area. To this day, Henry considers himself a very lucky fellow. He was just a few bullets short of being mutilated, hacked to death by that angry mob, and dismembered, a lovely little custom in this area of the world.

STREET SURVIVAL LESSONS

1) *Spot crime patterns.* Henry hiked in an area that was the scene of repeated ambushes, the horrid results of which were shown on nightly TV. Henry was warned that a favorite trick of the ambushers was to turn road signs, yet he seemed oblivious to the possibility that it could actually happen to him.

2) *Never hike alone.* Always hike with at least one other person. This is not only for making attacks upon your person less likely. Hiking accidents occur, and having a fellow hiker could spell the difference between life or death.

3) *Use a good map.* Never go into an unknown area without a good road map that you have studied well beforehand. Henry should have realized instantly that something was wrong and that he was hiking too far down an unpaved road. If he had studied his map before he set out and had it on him, it would have been obvious. He was too sure of himself.

4) *Be alert to abnormal behavior.* Sometimes people telegraph their thoughts through seemingly simple actions or lack of them. Be aware of this. Even when those teenagers didn't wave, but instead smiled malevolently, Henry still moved blissfully forward into uncharted territory. This is not to

say a friendly smile and wave should have fooled him, but their attitude clearly telegraphed a warning. Henry didn't pick up that warning or any other one. More examples: The village did not have a single soul in its streets. No cars were moving. No one was at a door, a window. It seemed deserted. He should have asked himself why. He should have turned back and got out of there. He didn't. He kept on, moving deeper into a potential ambush situation.

5) *Take cover.* Once engaged by the mob, he did react properly by jumping behind some rocks. This and having a good gun and plenty of ammo on him saved his life.

6) *Conserve ammunition.* Don't waste ammunition. Always fire semiauto or with short, controlled bursts whenever possible. Firing long bursts was very wasteful of precious ammunition. It could have cost Henry his life.

7) *Shoot to kill.* If necessary, don't hesitate to shoot to kill. In this case, shooting to scare rather than kill was a tactical decision based on his fear of acting against the law in his use of lethal force. He was wrong. Henry was very lucky it all worked out.

8) *Notify someone of your route.* When hiking through isolated areas, notify someone of your route, time of departure, and estimated time of arrival. This includes the authorities whenever possible. Henry was lucky the Border Police heard shots and investigated.

Today, Henry uses and studies a road map. He watches the news media with a trained eye and ear, looking for anything that could shift the odds in his favor as he hikes throughout the land of

Israel. He travels with at least one other hiker. He alerts the military of his route. He has survived an ambush and now has made street survival training a part of his life. He now has 12 Uzi magazines plus a Glock 19 along with eight loaded magazines all on him if needed. He admits he still wakes up at night in a sweat, hearing those screaming, yelling, cursing voices.

SPOTTING COVER

Forewarned is forearmed. Cover is usually all around us. It pays to develop an eye for it so that if you are ambushed your brain automatically ignites and your muscles spring into gear, placing you behind suitable cover. Henry did practice taking cover when he shot in practice. He did react instantly to the ambush and instead of trying to outrun his attackers, took cover.

Unfortunately, Hollywood westerns have made many people think that the way to react to a confrontation is to draw one's gun and walk down the center of the street, facing one's enemy man to man. Such pictures in the brain can get one killed.

Taking cover is a basic tool of street survival. Practice taking it as much as you practice drawing your weapon. Your weapon and cover should go hand in hand. From behind suitable cover you can control the field of the street battle. You control the situation, even against seemingly insurmountable odds.

One has only to remember the epic Battle of Thermopylae, where a handful of Spartan Greeks held off hundreds of thousands of Persians and their allies. The Spartans defended a narrow pass from behind the cover of their shields. The enemy was forced to fight the battle on the Spartans' terms. The numerically superior invading army was forced to channel its forces into a narrow battlefield. This won time for the Greek nation states and saved their independence. Well-thought-out cover saved the day against vastly superior forces and altered the course of history.

A fire hydrant is almost impossible to penetrate. A shallow blip on the street, such as a low curb, can afford suitable cover when nothing else exists. Telephone and light poles give readily available cover, and they are everywhere. Old-fashioned street mailboxes can stop many types of bullets, but trash cans do not. They look like cover, but unless filled with bricks, can be easily penetrated in a shoot-out.

Learn to think cover. Make lists of possible cover. Learn which items look like cover but are really death traps in the street. Test what effect cover will have on the bullets you carry.

Test-Fire against Cover

I remember being on the shooting range when the commander of the Israeli Armored Corps paid me a visit. We were out in the desert at the time, and I had invited him to drop by when he was in the area with an eye toward having him drop off the .38 Enfield pistol, an armored corps handgun left over from British Mandatory times. When his jeep pulled up, I proceeded to fire a cylinder full of .38 S&W bullets at a metal barrel. He emerged wide-eyed as he saw the lead smears on that dented barrel. Not one bullet had penetrated even one side of that barrel. A picture was certainly worth a thousand words. His eyes were opened as to the limitations of the .38 S&W bullet for military use in a way that no amount of talking could do. Against that bullet even a rusted old barrel could act as cover.

I then fired 9mmP and .45 ACP military ball at the barrel, and he examined the holes. Nothing further needed to be said. You also may be surprised when you view the effects of the bullets you carry on target. Remember—better to learn the facts of life on the range than in the street.

STREET SURVIVAL LESSON

1) *Know the difference between cover and conceal-*

ment. Know which items commonly on the street provide suitable cover against a host of bullets. If the cover you choose won't stop a pistol bullet, it certainly will not stop bullets fired from long guns.

....

Case Study: Lights Out

It was a time of war in 1973, and orders had been given for all lights to be out or behind cover so as to keep the city dark. Kurt and Ami walked up to an Arab cafe in the old city section of east Jerusalem. I moved against the wall across from them, covered by the blackness of the night, pistol in hand. Suddenly, the stillness was broken by approaching footsteps. He stopped and lit a cigarette. The flames illuminated me in the dark doorway. I'll never forget his astonished face as he hastily put out that match. Then I heard someone call out my name. I saw Kurt and Ami enter the cafe. I followed, being careful to stay far enough behind to see everything and anyone around them.

It was something out of a B movie of what most Westerners think the Mideast looks like: crowded . . . noisy

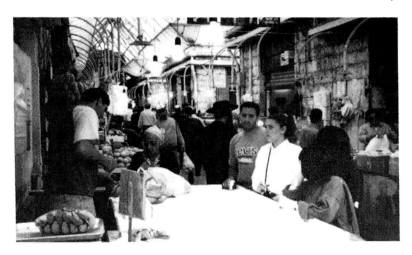

A SMALL SIDE STREET IN THE SHUK: An ideal place for the laying of bombs. An alert Israeli public has thwarted numerous bomb attempts.

. . . heavy smoke . . . men with the tips of the hollow cords of "bubble pipes" in their mouths, cords attached to bottles where tobacco burned in little metal trays on top . . . lots of card playing and backgammon games.

I moved against the wall as Kurt and Ami moved through the less-than-friendly crowd, checking IDs. Kurt asked, "Are there any Picassos here," as he had them show them their hands. He was checking to see if any tell-tale paint smears were there, a sure-fire way of knowing that the owner of such hands had painted a slogan calling for the murder of Israelis.

Kurt was a master at spotting terrorists. Only the day before (or was it just one day? Patrolling around the clock for days made it all seem like an endless maze), he had asked one cafe client to roll up his sleeve. He picked him out of a hundred men. That one guy. He was a particularly stupid terrorist, since he had the emblem of El Seiqua, the Syrian-based terror organization, tattooed on his arm. Kurt was good at his job—the best. We threw the tattooed guy in the back of a Border Police jeep, and I was assigned to ride shotgun with him. Let me tell you, if looks could kill, he could have killed me on the spot.

Anyway, getting back to that cafe with all those potential "Picassos." Kurt and Ami walked out while I remained standing at that wall, using it as most welcome back cover. Suddenly, one of the waiters jumped around and began mimicking Kurt in a most unfriendly manner, flipping and waving his hands back and forth in a very hilarious way. His back was to me, so he couldn't see me enjoying his act. He just couldn't figure out why his friends didn't laugh until he turned to see me against that wall, smile on my face, .45 in hand. He kept on waving his hands, but, changing the gyrations to that of circulating the air, he chimed out, "Boy, it's hot in here!" What an idiot. I just didn't have the heart to arrest him and, still grinning, walked past the somber faces of the patrons of the cafe, who looked quite relieved that everything had passed without incident.

Once outside, Kurt reprimanded me for not arresting the

guy. I disagreed, claiming the mimic was quite talented and lamenting the fact that Kurt and Ami missed it all. Anyway, the moral of the story is, use back cover; it has its place in potentially unpleasant situations.

....

STREET SURVIVAL LESSONS

1) *Use dark shadows and back cover to your advantage.* Outside the cafe, I was almost immune to ambush because I used the wall to cover my back and moved into the darkness. The same tactic worked in the cafe.

2) *Guard with weapon in hand.* Whenever possible, especially when the situation lends itself to the act, have your weapon out.

3) *Be just and fair.* Have a sense of humor. You don't always have to escalate every situation. In this case, I still believe Kurt was wrong and I was right in not arresting the waiter. As long as he stopped his little act when he saw me, he in effect bowed to the power and honor of the law. Arresting him would have been wrong and would have hardened the crowd. Never do a needless injustice; it only fuels the flames.

....

Case Study: Attempted Mugging in Manhattan

Many years ago, I paid a visit to the "Big Apple." I had not been in New York City in years and decided to stay at a hotel off Times Square. Such an idea had been quite acceptable in the 1950s, and I naively thought that was still the case.

Being an avid connoisseur of the so-called "Greasy Spoon Diner," I left my hotel in search of such as establishment. Fried eggs and home-fried potatoes served with a good cup of brewed coffee is my idea of living it up. It was a bitterly freezing cold night, and I pulled my jacket hood tighter as I walked through a snowstorm along a lonely side street toward the welcoming blinking neon lights of an all-night diner.

I was passing by a pitch dark alley when I suddenly felt an arm attempting to get me into a head lock. I instinctively bent low and jammed my elbow into my attacker's solar plexus in a series of hard blows. He fell back onto the street, hitting his head on the pavement with a resounding crack. I prepared to continue with him, when two of New York's finest, who had been viewing the encounter from inside an empty store, ran out and scooped up the somewhat dazed unsuccessful mugger as if he was a pile of refuse and they were a forklift truck. As they did this, they smiled at me and we exchanged waves as they took him into the alley and proceeded to pound him into the ground. The whole thing took no more than a few seconds.

I proceeded to the diner and over a cup of coffee and a blue plate special of fried eggs and potatoes, mulled over what had happened. I realized that the cops being in that storefront was a real stroke of luck, something out of the ordinary. What really bothered me was how that damn mugger got the jump on me? Even though I survived, I had a gnawing feeling in my stomach that I had really messed up. I was lucky I was still in one piece. I came to some conclusions by the time I had finished a slice of apple pie.

PREVENT ATTACKS BY BODY LANGUAGE

I have, over the years, become more and more convinced that I invited the incident in Manhattan by not telegraphing any deterrent body language. I was bent over, huddled against the cold wind. Had I stood erect, facing ahead, chances are the mugger would have waited for a more inviting target.

Body language is a most primitive form of deterrent that can work in your favor. Animals display it when they are challenged by other creatures. A dog will growl, bare its teeth, and expand its body by fanning its hair out. A cat will hiss and do the same. Body language, in this its most primitive form, is a manner of speaking without language, warning an enemy that you are not an easy target, that you are ready, willing, and able to defend yourself if attacked. It telegraphs that you are getting ready to inflict real harm on your adversary.

With human beings, body language takes on a much more subtle nature, at least in its early stages. How you carry yourself, how you move, all this signals that you are either in control and not afraid or the opposite. The primitive language of the jungle is alive in the urban jungles of today.

Case Study: Body Language at 3 A.M.

It was the time of the Yom Kippur War, and a blackout was in force, making the dark alleys of the old city section of Jerusalem even more foreboding.

Kurt and I were out alone that night when we approached a block of apartments in a courtyard to make what we considered a routine arrest. Of course, deep inside we knew there was really no such thing as routine. Only streaks of moonlight illuminated Kurt as he knocked on a large wooden door. The door creaked open and an Arab woman screamed that her husband wouldn't go.

Kurt pushed past her, collared the man, and shoved him out into the courtyard, when, all at once, as if on cue, shouting neighbors streamed around Kurt, forming a tight circle.

At this, I slipped off the thumb safety of my .45 auto and readied myself for what I believed was going to be one hell of a situation. Then I saw something that has since stuck in my mind as a prime example of what the Israelis call "chutzpah" (unmitigated gall). Kurt stuck his swagger stick under his arm and proceeded to inform all and sundry that he was an officer of the law, that the man was under arrest, and that anyone who blocked his way would be arrested. At this, Kurt slowly pushed through the hostile crowd, making eye contact with each person standing in front of him. In what seemed like an eternity, the crowd slowly opened a path for him and he pushed the suspect in my direction.

When he was close enough, I stepped out, .45 at the ready. The crowd spotted me. It grew very silent as the pistol slowly arched across their line of vision. At this, the hostile crowd melted away. The courtyard was dark and silent once more.

As we moved down a dark alley, suspect in hand, Kurt looked at me and smiled: "I have to admit that was about the wildest collar I ever made. Tell me, would you have shot if they suddenly attacked?"

"Kurt," I confided, "I would have done a .45 tap dance across the chest of anyone who even rubbed a hair on your chinny-chin-chin." He laughed as we moved down that dark alley. The suspect gave us no sweat, all the time glancing at the .45.

Interview with Kurt

Kurt's was the superb and professional use of body language at its best. He did not have to shout or wave his pistol about. Rather, he gave a much more potent message with body language. I questioned him about this:

E.S.: What were the body language tricks you used that night to ward off a riot?

K: Well, for openers, I stood ramrod straight, walking with a firm stride. Bending over even slightly is a form of submission. Walking in a hesitant manner telegraphs fear and weakness of will. All this is picked up by predators, be they one suspect or a crowd of potential rioters. Weakness excites predators. They smell it, just as a shark smells blood. It's the trigger mechanism for mayhem.

E.S.: You once mentioned that looking people in the eye is a form of body language. Could you elaborate?

K: Eye contact with strangers is something people avoid. It makes people nervous, as it is considered a type of intimacy. However, when someone on the street threatens you, it is critical that you look that person straight in the eye. This also goes for police officers making an arrest or questioning a suspect in the street. Looking directly at whoever you are speaking to gives out a subliminal message of your strength.

E.S.: I remember when we patrolled the narrow streets of the Casbah, you mentioned for us never to break eye contact with those individuals staring out at us from doorways, etc.

K: Exactly. Whenever you have someone stare at you and you stare back and they still keep on staring, that person is not acting in a manner [in which] normal people act out in the street. This is especially true when they are staring at an officer of the law in uniform. People tend to look away when you look at them. When they don't, chances are they are challenging you with body language, testing you by what nature considers a belligerent act, the way predators stare at their potential victims. Staring is considered a warning in the animal world and usually results in the potential victim running for its life. Because of this phenomenon, you must outstare the person who is staring at you. Do not break off eye contact. Make the other person lower his eyes or look away. Then you have won the battle of body language. Of course, as you always like to point out, there are no absolutes in street survival, and there are some predators out there who desire conflict at any price. You therefore have to be prepared to use force if necessary. That evening in Jerusalem, body language worked, avoiding conflict. Another night it might have failed and a riot would have broken out.

E.S: What about speaking?

K: My rule is, say it simple, say it short, and above all else, say it in a firm, calm manner that clearly signals you are in control and not fearful or confused. You telegraph [that] you know exactly what you want and you are going to get it. You are not bluffing, and you will not back down. I don't care if you are pissing in your pants, you must never have even an eyelash quiver. Use all the tools of body language at your disposal just as professionally as you use your guns in deadly confrontations. With such an attitude, you will sometimes find that you will not have to use force of any kind. Body language will have done the job. But be prepared to instantly use force if needed.

STREET SURVIVAL LESSONS

1) *Never, never let your guard down.* Bad weather is no excuse for letting your guard down. Some street predators favor such weather as that snowstorm in Manhattan to do their hunting in.

2) *Look formidable.* Deterrence works. Don't cancel the beneficial effect of looking formidable. My being all bundled up that way in Manhattan canceled out any deterrent effect my body language would have had on the hunting street predator. Instead, what he saw was a huddled over, seemingly easy target waiting to be pounced on. In effect, I had acted as unwilling bait, attracting rather than repelling my attacker.

3) *Explosive reaction.* When attacked, do the unexpected. My instinctive and explosive reaction to the attack caught my street mugger totally by surprise. He was thrown back, completely off balance, and fell to the street, dazed. I never knew if he had a weapon because those two cops intervened. Pure, unadulterated luck on my part. I shudder to think what would have happened if he had plunged a knife into my back or pulled a gun.

   The incident was really my first taste of what had so drastically changed for the worse out there in the streets of New York City since the days when you could almost walk anywhere without being assaulted. I vowed to capitalize on my foolish luck and never to be caught napping again.

4) *Look someone in the eye.* Never lower your eyes when you are speaking, giving orders, or when someone challenges you. Lowering the eyes is a sign of submission and can invite attack.

5) *Never be the first to break eye contact.* Make the other fellow lower or turn his eyes away.

6) *Speak in a confident manner.* Garbled, hesitant speech is a sign of weakness and invites, rather than repels, street predators. When facing down a crowd, or anyone for that matter, don't shout or act like you are losing self-control. Speak in a firm, clear, cool manner. It is much more awesome.

7) *Backup partner.* Always try to work with at least one backup. "One ranger, one riot" is good. But "two rangers, one riot" is even better.

....

Case Study: The Blue Knife Murder

A recent case of cold-blooded murder has much to teach us about street survival. Haim Darina, a staff sergeant in the Israeli army, was stabbed to death by an Arab as he sipped a soft drink outside a cafe adjacent to the Nahal Õz crossing, an area some 20 yards outside the perimeter fence of the Gaza Strip. Darina was murdered by Iyad Salim Arir of Gaza City, a student at the Islamic College there. Arir was subsequently overpowered by Zvi Sa'ar, an Israeli kibbutz member who worked at the cafe. Arir was arrested and turned over to the Israeli General Security Service.

Darina, 41, had just called his mother, who was concerned about his safety, and told her, "Mom, I'm fine and there's nothing to worry about." Other soldiers who were near him left the cafe, and Darina sat alone on a bench in the sun, sipping his drink. It was then that Arir rushed him and stabbed him in the throat, grabbing his M16 rifle. Darina staggered a few yards, collapsed, and bled to death.

Sa'ar, the Israeli cafe employee, saw what happened, pushed a burglar alarm button, and then charged at the terrorist, jumping on him just as he cocked the M16 and pointed it at the Israeli.

"I tipped the table on him and knocked him to the floor. I kicked the weapon away and lay on top of him until the army came," Sa'ar said.

IDF sources claimed that the quick reaction of the cafe employee probably saved many lives, as the terrorist planned to open fire on everyone in sight.

Arir was armed with a knife whose handle was a blue plastic tube. A second half of the blue plastic tube covered an 8-inch knife blade. The terrorist had passed through the checkpoint a couple of hours before and apparently had not been stopped or searched. He then loitered outside the cafe, waiting for the opportunity to catch a soldier alone. When Darina filled the bill, Arir struck.

During the investigation, Sa'ar admitted to having a licensed handgun, which he had left at home because he did not feel he needed it at work. Nothing bad ever had happened at work before.

STREET SURVIVAL LESSONS

1) *Never totally rely on others for your security.* Darina saw the soldiers at the checkpoint and may have believed he was safe. He was not. The terrorist had somehow moved through the checkpoint without being searched properly. This is believable, since thousands of Arabs do this around the clock, making real security checks almost impossible, as they go into Israel proper to work.

2) *Danger knows no borders.* Since he was on what was considered the safe side of the crossing, Sa'ar and Darina were relaxed. Sa'ar saw the terrorist, Arir, loitering for hours, and yet did not question him.

3) *Don't leave your handgun at home.* Sa'ar's "all is well" attitude had him leave his handgun at home. He now says he will carry it to work.

4) *Innocent-looking objects can be deadly.* The blue tube in Arir's hand did not look suspicious enough for anyone at the border checkpoint or the cafe to question.

5) *Never lose vigilance.* Always have your weapon ready. This error cost Darina his life. Sa'ar showed courage as he attacked the terrorist with his bare hands. Unfortunately, if he had been more vigilant, he might have been able to challenge the terrorist earlier.

6) *Study criminal attacks.* Don't just read about them; study them. Learn to decipher the main teaching points to be learned so that you do not fall victim to them. What happened to Staff Sgt. Darina had happened dozens of times before. It had been written about in the press and seen on the TV news. His tragic death could have been avoided.

STREET DOGS

Probably the most underutilized weapon for street survival is the dog. For street survival, it is imperative that your dog look like he means business. This means something of the size of a German shepherd or rottweiler. After all, deterrence is the best defense of all. The most vicious small dog in the world is still an unproven commodity until he actually gets into action. The deterrent value of a large dog is something you do not want to neglect. It's a vital first barrier that may ward off trouble.

Besides coming in different sizes, dogs come with different levels of street effectiveness. Here in the Mideast, there is an old wives' tale about black dogs being more frightening to criminals and terrorists than dogs of any other color. Don't you believe such things. These theories are usually just that— unproven theories that are completely meaningless out in the street. In the street, old wives' tales can get you killed. I remember seeing two black dogs tied to a house. Inside, their master had been robbed and brutally murdered.

One of the problems with having a dog out on the street with you is that it must be leashed and muzzled. A uniformed police officer does take the muzzle off of his canine when he works, but a civilian has a real problem. Walking an unmuzzled dog in most cities is breaking the law. Not to mention the lawsuit you would face if your dog were to bite someone passing by. The technical problem faced by the dog owner on the street is one based on his assessment of the threat level he faces. Of course, if one sees trouble up ahead, one can unmuzzle the dog. But in doing this, two problems arise. First, one has to correctly assess that trouble does, in fact, exist. Second, one has to see the potential trouble. A muzzled dog is almost useless if you are ambushed and do not have the time to unmuzzle your canine friend. Fortunately, the dog may sense the ambush and potential trouble and warn you of it in advance. Still, leash and muzzle laws make the whole issue of dogs defending their law-abiding masters somewhat dicey. Fortunately, most street predators are not aware of the fact that the dog is "toothless" because of the muzzle and will still tend to avoid pedestrians with large dogs like the plague. What is needed is a really quick snap-off muzzle that is secure, yet fast to remove if one is attacked. To date, I have not seen such a design.

We will delve further into the use of our canine friends in Chapter 8.

....

STREET SURVIVAL LESSONS

1) *Bigger is better.* In this case, a large, powerful dog is a better deterrent to street attack than a small dog.

2) *Beware the dog muzzle.* A muzzled dog loses much of his actual counterattack capability.

3) *The dog is a street alarm.* A dog will usually sense danger before his master does.

4) *Old wives' tales can kill.* Don't believe in things that are talked about in the street but common sense tells you may be untrue. Black dogs may not scare anyone. (Big dogs aren't an old wives' tale; they do scare most people more than tiny ones.)

Case Study: Deadly Bait

Baum tells the following story of when he deliberately set himself up as bait for an ambush in the Casbah of Gaza City:

E.S.: Could you describe the time you deliberately did everything wrong in the hope that you would be attacked?

S.B.: There was a grenade attack that resulted in two young Israeli kids being blown up in the back seat of their family car as they were being driven past Gaza City. Because of this attack, Arik Sharon, myself, and some men I hand-picked went into Gaza to destroy the terror cells that had sprouted there in the late 1960s and early '70s as a result of our conquest following the Six-Day War.

I believed that Arab kids were the ones who were throwing grenades at passing Israeli civilian and military vehicles, but I was not interested in them. They could be bought for five Egyptian pounds a throw.

E.S.: So why not target them?

S.B.: What I was interested in was the adult who gave them the grenades and money. Once I got that adult ringleader, the network would fall apart. I had to set myself up as bait.

E.S.: Wasn't that risky? How could you know when the attack would be carried out? What if you didn't spot them in time?

S.B.: It was a calculated but necessary risk. I felt that the adult ringleader signaled the kid to throw the grenade. In the split second before he gave the signal, I had to kill that ringleader.

E.S.: How?

B: My plan was simple. I would be driven in an open military jeep through the crowded Gaza open-air marketplace at exactly the same time each day. I picked noon, when the sun was the hottest. I sat back in the jeep with my eyes closed, sunning myself. An open newspaper on my lap. One dumb officer.

E.S.: How long before something happened?

B: A week or so. We were pulling into the marketplace, and I noticed an Arab kid who looked nervous. He had something in his hand. A grenade. I watched his eyes. He looked up at a man standing above us on the flat roof. It was my target. I pulled a .30-caliber Mauser pistol from under the newspaper and let off a shot which hit the ringleader on the base of his chin and then blew the back of his head off. We got the kid. After that, no more grenades were thrown in Gaza. We then proceeded to destroy each and every terror cell in the Gaza Strip. We did. Peace and tranquillity came to Gaza. That lasted for 10 years . . . until the Intifada broke out. Unfortunately, Arik and I and our men (including you) were not allowed to handle it. It's gone on for seven years so far. A pity. We could have broken it in 72 hours.

STREET SURVIVAL LESSONS

1) *Beware repetitious patterns.* Criminals spot patterns of behavior. Such patterns, be they jogging, hiking, walking, taking money to the bank, etc., help them ambush their victims. Beware of doing the same task in exactly the same way every time.

   I was asked by a worried housewife whose husband had to bike through a particularly dangerous part of town every night at exactly the same time and route if I thought that was foolish. I told her she had answered her own question by even asking it. She was worried because it was indeed a foolish thing to do. A series of knife attacks had plagued the area. It was not a place for someone to travel through in a telltale pattern.

2)   *Intelligent bait.* Acting as intelligent bait is a good way of attracting and then destroying criminals bent on mayhem. However, this high-risk task is only a job for professionals.

Chapter Seven

In the Vehicle

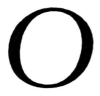One of the most grievous errors made by amateurs in street survival is the lack of having a route plan before driving a vehicle into an unknown area. We spoke about the use of good maps in the chapter entitled "In the Street." It is imperative that you have not only a good map but a mental picture of the area and planned route. This means memorizing landmarks that can be called to mind instantly if seen or missed. You should be absolutely aware at all times as to your location on that mental map. The less you have to stop the car to check a map the better. A vehicle pulled over to the shoulder of the road provides street predators with an easy mark. On the other hand, trying to drive while you check a road map is a formula for getting into accidents. So plan that route in the quiet of your living room and easy chair, not out there in the street.

THE FLASHLIGHT TECHNIQUE

Approaching and entering your vehicle makes you vulnerable to attack. Criminals like to lie in wait inside their victims' vehicles or hide behind them like some spider waiting for prey. At night, if your car is outside, try to park under lights. A locked garage is even better, though it is still no guarantee that someone hasn't gained entry. Whether parking inside or out, always approach your car with your keys and flashlight (a small thin one is preferred) in your weak hand. Your right hand is then free to draw your handgun or, if desired, have the handgun already in it.

Illuminate the car's exterior and then its interior. Never enter a dark car. If all looks well, transfer the end of the flashlight to your mouth. That's right, your mouth. This is an excellent little street trick that works like a charm because in this position the flashlight illuminates whatever you look at. Hear a sound to your right or left? Turn and its beam follows your eyes. Look down at the lock. You see it. All the time your strong hand remains free to work the handgun, while your weak hand opens the door of your car. (This technique works anywhere, including when opening the front door of your house.)

The flashlight technique is the correct answer when you have to juggle keys, flashlight, and handgun at the same time. The added bonus is having the flashlight beam follow your eyes.

BOOBY TRAPS

Since this book is for worldwide publication, it is pertinent to speak about something that is not uncommon in some parts of the world—namely, booby-trapped vehicles. One does not necessarily have to be a VIP to face this danger. Terrorists are increasingly using booby-trapped vehicles as a means of creating mass death and destruction. The vehicle filled with high explosives has become the calling card of terrorists. However, you sometimes can spot booby-trapped vehicles by knowing a few tricks of the trade.

The Mirror Technique
Before you check for the abnormal, it is important to have a mental picture of what normal looks like. Get to know what

your car looks like when viewed from underneath. The best way to do this is when it is on a lift in the garage. Simply crawling underneath a parked vehicle does not really afford one a proper overall view of the area and actually provides a very distorted, segmented picture that may be hard to imprint on the mind. A good diagram of the underside of the vehicle is provided in some car manuals and is a very helpful guide to follow.

A very easy way to check under your car for any unwanted items is by the simple expedient of attaching a pocket mirror to a long stick (preferably a curved one for more convenience) and running it under the car as you look for telltale wires that seem out of order.

A second area to know well and check thoroughly is underneath the hood, especially the electrical parts attached to the battery and engine. Bombers like to use the car's own ignition system for closing the electrical gap to detonate an explosive device. Knowing your vehicle's electrical system is critical to spotting any bomb connected to it.

A third area where bombs are sometimes hidden is underneath the car seats, especially the driver's seat. When in doubt, do not start your car but have it checked by a more expert person like an electrician. The procedure here in Israel is to call the bomb squad. Check if such a unit exists where you live. Bomb squads are the ultimate experts to handle the problem. Remember, better safe than sorry.

....

STREET SURVIVAL LESSONS

1) *Plan your route.* Have a good map of the route you intend to take and memorize landmarks. Try to have a mental picture so that you do not have to pull off the road to read the map or read it while in traffic.

2) *Park in a well-lit area.* When your car is parked for the night, be sure to have it under lights if outside or in a locked garage if left inside.

3)   *Weak hand holds keys and flashlight.* This leaves the strong hand free for shooting if necessary.

4)   *Flashlight technique.* Using your teeth to hold the end of a small flashlight frees your gun hand and has the added bonus of directly illuminating whatever you are looking at.

5)   *Know your car.* Have a mental picture of the underside of your vehicle as well as its engine compartment.

6)   *Understand your car's electrical system.* You should place special emphasis on understanding your car's electrical system.

7)   *Mirror technique.* Use a mirror on a curved stick to see under the car.

8)   *Under car seats.* If suspicious, remember to check under your car's seats, a favorite hiding place for bombs.

9)   *Call an expert.* When in doubt, have an expert inspect the vehicle.

10) *Don't touch it.* Never attempt to physically touch or dismantle a bomb. This is a job for the experts. And even they can slip up. We've lost a few here over the years.

YOUR WAR CHARIOT

A vehicle has a lot of things going for it as far as street survival. It's fast, so it can get you away from a lethal confrontation. It does afford some limited protection from objects such as rocks, Molotov cocktails, or bullets. It is powerful enough to use as a weapon itself. However, there are some glaring weaknesses. The first is that visibility is very limited. Secondly, if alone, the driver has to control the vehicle besides protecting himself. This can prove to be a complicated juggling act at best. Third, if one has to fire at an enemy while driving, our traverse capability is severely limited. Fourth, most vehicles are road-bound and cannot move onto rough terrain. And finally, a standard vehicle (not armored) is like a tin foil barrier when fired upon and is easily perforated.

How can we overcome these basic deficiencies? How can we make the vehicle we are in a dangerous target for would-be ambushers—one they will avoid like the plague? How can these Israeli lessons be applied to the cities of North America and other parts of the globe?

Clean Windows

Let's begin with something as mundane as clean windows. The windows of your car should be washed and clean. It is absolutely amazing how much more one can see when the glass one is looking through is free of dust, sand, and bird or tree droppings. Get that glass clean so that you can spot minute details around you.

Primary Mirrors

Mirrors should be strategically placed. This includes an overhead one as well as large outside side mirrors in the areas of the right and left front doors.

Make sure these mirrors are not the kind that distort what you are seeing as is done by some of those panoramic designs. The ability to judge distance is critical, and primary mirrors that distort distance evaluation are dangerous.

Secondary Mirrors

With secondary mirrors—stress on the word secondary—that are placed to eliminate blind spots, some distortion can be allowed, though if you can fit secondary mirrors that give a panoramic view with little or no distortion, all the better.

These backup mirrors fill in the gaps the primary mirrors may have missed.

Rear Passenger Mirrors
Don't hesitate to include mirrors for the passengers in the rear of your vehicle. This is almost never done in thinking about vehicle security. Neglecting to do this is a mistake. You cannot have too many mirrors in your vehicle that act as extra eyes.

Off-Road Capability
The ability to move off a paved road into a field during a vehicle ambush is not one that should be taken lightly. Using oversized tires (my Volvo passenger car sports such tires) should improve a passenger car's ability to go cross-country in such an emergency. Putting in an improved suspension system is a good idea, along with an extra strong front bumper to enable even a passenger vehicle to burst through some types of man-made barriers or even small trees. Being road-bound is a definite hindrance to street survival, and anything that allows your vehicle to leave the road can only improve your chances.

Extra Equipment Options
If you live in an area that is riot-prone, it may be prudent to add or change things on your vehicle that take such problems into consideration. Israel has been a very practical testing ground for finding solutions to this problem, one that runs the spectrum from stones to bullets aimed at cars.

High-Impact Glass
Rioters around the world like to use weapons of opportunity, and the common stone fits the bill quite nicely. More advanced rioters use Molotov cocktails. Any of these missiles, when they are thrown through the air and impact on a fast-moving car, can cause havoc inside a vehicle. In Israel, a new special clear plastic addition glued to car windows has reduced injury to driver and passengers in areas prone to

stone-throwing. These have been found to withstand rocks the size of baseballs, though heavy boulders are another matter, especially when the velocity of such missiles is increased by the forward movement of the vehicle.

Stones have killed people here. A few victims are still "alive," living out their lives attached to life-support systems. Anyone who tells you stones aren't weapons is a damn liar. Stones are deadly. They have probably killed as many people in warfare over many thousands of years as any of our modern weapons.

Heavy Wire Screening

Another option on vehicles that must drive through a gauntlet of rocks, iron bars, and Molotov cocktails is the addition of a heavy wire screen to the front window. Some of my friends in Jerusalem have placed them on their front car windows and claim it has the added benefit of making it quite impossible for car thieves to steal front wipers.

The heavy wire screen will usually defeat almost any size rock that can be thrown by a human being. Drivers using such additions claim that you soon get used to them and visibility does not suffer. Of course, these additions will not stop bullets nor certain types of projectiles that resemble bullets. I remember driving to a shooting tournament with a friend of mine who cautioned me that we were approaching a very dangerous village. It seems his friend had traveled the same road only the week before, and some Arab teenager had fired a ball bearing at his car from a slingshot. The ball bearing went through the front window, took out the overhead mirror, and continued out the rear window. Needless to say, such a missile would have had the same effect on the driver's head as a rifled slug fired from a 12-gauge shotgun.

Beware Inflammable Car Roofs

The use of highly inflammable rubber or plastic tarpaulins as roofs, draped across the tops of open vehicles, is definitely not recommended if you live in an area where rioters throw Molotov cocktails. A wonderfully brave Israeli officer

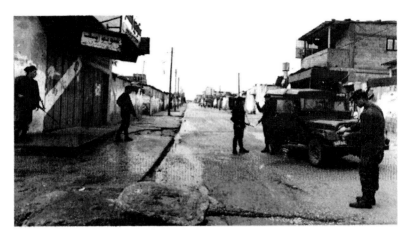

ISRAELI BORDER POLICE JEEP: An Arab village that has been placed under curfew. Notice the metal screens on the Jeep's windows and the hard roof.

appeared on national TV after his jeep was hit by a Molotov cocktail. It was in the early days of the Intifada. The flaming gasoline instantly melted the rubber tarpaulin over the officer's head, and the burning molten mass fell down onto him. His face was gone. Most Israeli jeeps now have solid roofs.

Sirens

A siren is another good idea. Having a switch next to the driver that activates a very loud siren (for civilian vehicles) could have a very unexpected and demoralizing effect on someone who does not expect it. The use of noise as a psychological weapon in warfare goes back to the dawn of human history. Having an electrical siren is only a method of upgrading a proven tool, a battle cry of the car.

STREET SURVIVAL LESSONS

1) *Clean windows*. Have clean windows when setting out on the road. What you can't see can hurt you.

2)   *Mirrors.* The use of primary and secondary mirrors is critical to giving you those needed extra eyes.

3)   *Wide-track tires.* Wide-track tires should be explored for vehicular use since they add to your cross-country capabilities.

4)   *High-impact windows.* High impact additions to your car's windows is a must if you drive through riot-prone areas.

5)   *Heavy wire screens.* Wire screening is another option for window protection from heavier rocks.

6)   *Nonflammable car roofing.* Avoid meltdown caused by Molotov cocktails landing on inflammable car roofs.

7)   *Siren.* A siren (when legal) placed on a civilian vehicle is simply upgrading the basic time-honored use of a sudden loud noise, the battle cry used to confuse and demoralize an attacker. It can also alert others that you are under attack.

YOUR VEHICLE IS A LETHAL WEAPON

Most people don't realize that the most powerful weapon they will ever control in their lives is the family car. Talk about momentum or kinetic energy, the family car makes a handheld weapon pale by comparison. Yet, most of us, even when faced by a potentially deadly attack, will do the exact opposite of what we should do when seated behind the wheel.

Case Study: Boulder Attack
A few years back I saw a classic example of someone in a car attacked by someone wielding a massive boulder. It was a road outside of Kiryat Arba, an Israeli town in southern

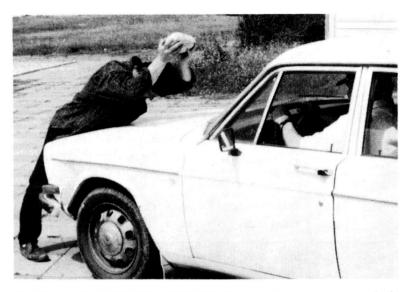

YOUR CAR IS A LETHAL WEAPON: Never hesitate to use it as such if attacked.

Israel. An Israeli was driving his car toward Jerusalem when a rioter rushed into the street, a huge boulder held above his head. Now I'm not saying it was fishy that a TV cameraman just happened to be there (these type of photo opportunities also occur in Israel where foreign TV cameramen are accused of staging and paying for such attacks) and filmed the incident in living color as the attacker plunged the boulder through the car's front window.

The driver reacted as he would have reacted when faced with a pedestrian in his path: he braked and turned to avoid hitting him. The car stopped and the driver slumped forward, bleeding profusely. He was lucky; his assailant ran away. If the perp had pressed forward with the attack, we would have seen a murder rather than grievous bodily harm on the TV news.

Driver Retraining

Good scenario planning and retraining can change our inner thoughts on vehicle control. One of the hardest things you would ever have to do in reacting to such an attack is the exact opposite of what you've done all your life—namely, gun the engine and run over your attacker with all the tons of raw energy your car possesses. To do such a thing means relearning the mental conditioning of a lifetime—no easy task. But it can be done if you practice doing it as part of your street survival training.

The idea is to cultivate the image in your mind of someone attacking you rather than crossing in front of your vehicle. The way to do this is to set up a target (the type seen on some shooting ranges) of someone holding a knife or gun and then practice turning your vehicle into that picture rather than away from it. This must be done along with practicing with friendly targets, much like you practice target selection in a shooting scenario. In time, you will do it as a matter of course, and you just might react correctly to save your life.

STREET SURVIVAL LESSONS

1) *Cars are lethal weapons*. Understand that your vehicle is a deadly weapon, probably the most powerful one you will ever control. View it as such. Scenario plan and retrain using your vehicle as a lethal weapon if you are under attack.

2) *Target selection*. Realistic training with your vehicle means using friendly and unfriendly targets as you would your firearms. Practice target selection as you drive toward these targets.

The Lone Armed Driver

Driving alone in isolated areas this day and age is a mistake, but sometimes an unavoidable one. Driving alone in areas that exhibit a high risk of vehicular attacks (as indicated on the map you use to chart such activities) is insanity and must be avoided at all costs. Unfortunately, the lone driver must sometimes face even this high-risk situation.

When you are driving, it is best to have a handgun available. Rifles, submachine guns, and shotguns are usually suited for use by the driver when the vehicle is stopped. For top efficiency, they necessitate the use of two hands to bring them into play when the vehicle is moving, an impossible task for the driver to accomplish.

One-handed fire can be done with submachine guns but is still somewhat of a difficult exercise. Jonathan has fired his Uzi from his pick-up truck and admits that the task is not a simple one since the weight of the Uzi makes good control somewhat difficult. He admits to slowly coming around to my suggestion of using handguns—and only handguns—for this task when driving a vehicle. Behind the wheel, a handgun is the primary weapon of choice—a gun for the hand, not hands.

WEAPON AND AMMO STORAGE

I have always been a firm believer in the axiom that only the weapons and ammunition you have on you are guaranteed to be there in an emergency. This is especially true in vehicles. Bailing out of the vehicle while under fire is not the time to be grabbing ammunition or weapons from where they are stored. What you have on you is more than likely what you'll have to work with. Never count on that weapon and ammo sitting in the trunk; you may not be able to get to them. The same goes for placing such items in the car's glove compartment or in a briefcase. Likewise for what you have near but not on you. Never leave a handgun or extra ammo on the seat next to you. They will almost certainly crash to the floor and rattle away under your seat if you are forced to accelerate suddenly or slam on the brakes. Long guns are less susceptible to this, though they are best held in a fast break clamp.

Once again, this makes a good case for the handgun, a lethal weapon that is always on you. In a car, the best weapon for the driver is the handgun, head and shoulders over any other firearm. The handgun excels in the very close-quarter and restrained environment of a vehicle. It works in narrow spaces and was the weapon of choice for the American "tunnel rats" in Vietnam.

High-Capacity Magazine
In the vehicle is where the use of an extra high-capacity magazine is not only a viable option but excels. Hanging on to the steering wheel, changing a magazine, and reloading a revolver are exercises that don't mix very well. Of course, the use of a backup handgun will probably give one all the ammo needed for such a situation. Still, having a handgun filled with more than six to eight bullets would be a comfort.

For those who have the standard-capacity semiauto such as the 1911, there are special extra-long magazines that hold from 11 to 16 rounds of the big .45 bullet. However, be careful and thoroughly test them with your carry ammo to make sure they function as well as advertised. Reports say all do not do as well as claimed.

I have found the extra length in the street is not handy and may even get in the way of a properly timed draw, but in the car they work reasonably well, and their virtues far outweigh their faults.

Standard high-capacity handguns such as the Para-Ordnance or Caspian Arms, which already have double-column magazines with 14 rounds in them plus one up the spout, do the trick nicely. The same for Glocks in .45 and 9mmP.

Driver's Window: Open or Closed?
The driver's window should usually be open so that the handgun can be brought into play efficiently. Fumbling for a window button or knob is not the easiest thing to do when under attack. However, there are two problems with keeping the window open when driving. One is driving in rain or snow. In such weather, an open window may not be acceptable to many. This is an individual choice. Personally, I keep the window wide open, deeming my health to be more in jeopardy from bullets than from rain or snow. However,

there is one exception to this rule, and that is when I am driving at slow speed through a potentially hostile crowd. I spoke about this problem here as early as 1971 and received few takers for the idea of closing the window in this situation. The idea was generally rejected as very impractical if one didn't have an air conditioner and a heat wave was on. This skepticism soon changed.

Case Study: Open Window Invites Attack

It was not long after I had voiced an opinion about the dangers of driving through a potentially hostile crowd at slow speed with the window open that an attack occurred which proved my point. A high-ranking Israeli Border Policeman was driving his car through an open marketplace when someone in the crowd walked past his car and dropped a hand grenade through the open window and onto his lap. The grenade fell to the floor and exploded, blowing off both his legs. I remember my phone ringing and the callers informing me of what had occurred. Of course, it was with no satisfaction that I learned of the tragedy and the correctness of my street survival reasoning. Sometimes dry theory becomes cruel reality. Keep that in mind when making a decision about your vehicle windows.

Plan out a scenario in your mind that tells you what type of dangers you may expect and take this into consideration when making a decision about those windows. Once again, there are no absolutes in personal security, only risks. You and only you must make an educated guess as to the potential worst-case scenario dangers you may face, knowing that nothing may happen for a thousand times and then the unexpected will occur just that once with irreversible consequences for you and your loved ones.

STREET SURVIVAL LESSONS

1) *Street survival tactics behind the wheel.* The principles of street survival apply when you are be-

hind the wheel—correct mind-set, full alertness, controlled anger, an explosive counterattack.

2) *Driver's handgun.* A driver must have a handgun ready for instant use if he is attacked. Long guns serve as primary weapons when the driver gets out of the vehicle.

3) *Weapons and ammo on you.* Only the weapons and ammunition on you can be counted on, since you may be forced to get out of the car at an instant's notice.

4) *Know the use of open or closed windows.* There are no easy rules for when to keep vehicle windows open or closed. Scenario planning can help you make up your mind when it is keyed into the potential threats you may face in a particular situation.

DRIVE-BY SHOOTERS TARGET THE DRIVER

We live in an age of crime, corruption, and terror. A good example is Los Angeles, where perhaps 200 street gangs, some with more than 200 members each, war over control of the drug trade. School yards become battlefields. Homes are blown up. Drive-by shootings turn streets and highways into butcher shops.

Israel is also experiencing such drive-by shootings, carried out by fanatical terrorists. The number of such attacks is definitely on the increase. Most of these shootings take place at night and on isolated roads, though daylight attacks on main roads are on the upturn. The killers especially like to drive stolen cars with Israeli license plates. They dress as Israelis, a tactic that helps lower the vigilance of their intended victims. They drive by, open up with submachine guns, then drive away at high speed.

Another tactic is to wait off the road and fire when the

victim's car is forced to slow down for a turn or obstacle in the road.

The innate ingenuity of the Israelis has begun to bring forth answers to thwart these murderous attacks.

The Frontal Ambush

If your attackers are in front of your vehicle, the best choice is sharply executing an evasive turnaround and speeding away from them. If that option is closed, you have two other choices. One would be to press down the accelerator and ram them at high speed—the explosive, angry, unexpected counterattack.

The other choice would be to brake and jump from the vehicle, using its engine, axle, or wheels as cover, or to roll off the road to better cover if available. From there you can engage your adversaries with fire.

Never stay in the vehicle, because once it stops, being behind the wheel does not afford proper cover nor the ideal of 360-degree trajectory of fire.

The Side Ambush

The ambush from the side can come from the side of the road or from a passing car. When I spent a short time as an outside consultant to an Israeli bus company, I saw a special range they had set up where their bus drivers were trained on how to respond to side attacks when they were at the wheel. The technique was to speed past the site of the attack while firing multiple shots from a pistol at the attackers so as to bring them down or have them dive for cover and break off their attack.

The problem with such a system is that it is inaccurate with regard to target selection and could possibly involve innocent casualties. But then again, it could be argued that a bus full of passengers, if not defended, could involve a much, much higher rate of fire directed against innocents.

Probably in no other confrontation are the scales so tipped in favor of the attacker as they are in drive-by shootings. Not only can the perpetrator pick the time and place of the attack, but he can sometimes speed away from the scene of the crime even before the alarm is sounded. This, of course, is why such tactics are becoming increasingly popular with criminals. Many murdered victims sit in bullet-riddled cars for hours before someone goes to see why a car is parked off the road or spots it turned over in some ditch.

The Rear Ambush
Eternal vigilance is the basis for street survival anywhere, and certainly out on the road. Being aware of the cars around, and especially behind you, is critical. Cars harboring drive-by killers tend to shadow their victim as they size up the opportune time to accelerate and pass, deluging their target with a hail of full-automatic fire.

The Brake Trick
Jonathan uses a technique for guarding against ambush by a suspicious car attempting to pass him on the road. As the car starts to pull up alongside, he slams on the brakes. Such a maneuver causes the passing car to fly past at high speed and results in the timing of any would-be drive-by killers to be thrown off balance. This maneuver, coupled with a ready Uzi or handgun, tips the odds more in his favor in that he uses the element of surprise to his advantage.

The Driver's-Side Window
Engaging targets from the driver's window while you hold the steering wheel in your hand borders on some sort of circus juggling act. For this problem, I have found the left hand to be the better choice even if one is right-handed. Firing left-handed out of the window gives one more flexibility and so helps achieve a greater field of fire.

Problems may arise with holster carry since a standard right-side holster makes such a left-handed quick draw nearly impossible, making it necessary to use the right hand for this task. A front cross draw (right or left side) with butt-forward carry will work nicely and is another reason I am becoming more and more enamored with this rig as I travel at night across the dark roads of Judea, Samaria, and Gaza, going to lecture and train settlers on how to survive their increasingly hostile environment.

The Passenger's-Side Window

Engaging targets out of the right front window while holding onto the steering wheel is another test of manual dexterity. Here the problem is the opposite for the driver, as the right hand is better suited to engage your enemy with. What to do? Again, I have solved this problem nicely by wearing a brace of front cross draw, butt forward .45 autos. However, if you have only one pistol and it is on your right side in the standard butt-rear position, you, of course, can

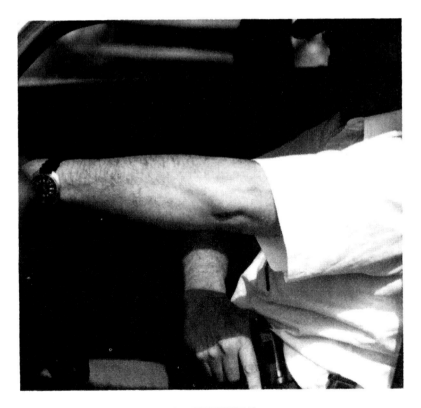

FRONT CROSS DRAW IN THE VEHICLE.

easily draw the pistol in the right hand to engage your targets in the right front window.

Once again, work on what's best for your particular situation and mode of carry. Whichever way you choose to engage targets from either of your windows, you must practice the maneuvers over and over if you are to carry them out smoothly and successfully.

The Side-Swipe Maneuver

The Hollywood favorite of slamming your car in a sideswipe maneuver into your attacker's vehicle may also be an excellent idea, provided your enemy is not sitting in a semi trailer or some other large truck.

The side-swipe technique works best against vehicles that are of the same or preferably less weight than the one you are driving. The chances of defeating a large truck are not high unless you are in an even larger one.

If your attacker is not expecting this maneuver, it may catch him off guard and allow you to regain control. Again, the principle of the explosive counterattack, a technique that usually works, is brought into play.

Case Study: Weapons Strategies of Ex-U.S. Cop, SWAT Team Member, and Ranger when Traveling Alone in PLO and Hamas Areas

Jonathan is a working board member, along with me, in the new Col. Mickey Marcus Institute, a nonprofit foundation dedicated to teaching and spreading the word about the principles of street survival. Baum acts as consultant to the board.

Mickey Marcus was a U.S. officer who came to Israel after World War II to help the fledgling Israeli state fight for its independence. Marcus was played by Kirk Douglas in the film *Cast a Giant Shadow*. John Wayne played his U.S. Army commander, both serving under the command of Gen. Dwight D. Eisenhower. I believe it is a most fitting name for our institute.

The three of us are also partners in The American-Israel Combat School, an Israeli facility dedicated to blending the very best techniques of combat, combat shooting, and street survival from the U.S. and Israel.

I interviewed Jonathan on the weapon he uses when driving alone in isolated areas.

E.S.: Jon, we've spoken of choice of firearms. What are you presently carrying and what do you plan to carry in the future?

J: My present primary weapon is the Uzi, though I hope to go to a short M16 at a later date. I carry the Uzi along with three loaded 9mmP magazines, staggering Winchester Black Talons along with IMI [Israel Military Industries] jacketed ball. It's the system I use because of the high cost of hollow-point ammo—here in Israel, about a buck a round.

My current back-up weapon is a Glock 21 with four extra loaded magazines. While I am partial to the Speer 200-grain hollowpoints, the so-called "flying ashtray" load, I also carry Winchester Black Talon, which is still legal here in Israel, along with Remington 230-grain military ball.

I plan to bring my Mini Uzi over from the States along with a slew of 9mm magazines for it and .45 magazines for the Glock.

E.S.: How many magazines?

J: Enough to take on a platoon yet still move with agility when I debus. In other words, I'll actually know when I put on my gun rig, load up, and train. Incidentally, I like the idea of a fanny pack you've been pushing for even more loaded magazines when isolation and ambush are possible. You and I know it can get mighty lonely out there on some back country road. Lots of extra ammo is not what one would call a luxury.

E.S.: What about a third weapon?

J: I now carry a Gerber boot knife but will eventually go for a second handgun in matching caliber if possible. As you know, Israeli gun laws forbid most of us peons from carrying matching calibers (you are a rare exception), so I may go for a Glock 19 in 9mmP, being careful not to mix up magazines as you caution us not to do. My ammo will be the same as for the Uzi.

Incidentally, after looking over the Applegate-Fairbairn Double-Edged Fighting Knife, I think I will purchase one for a fourth weapon that will also have a role as a utility knife for around the farm and for when I am on the road.

E.S.: What holster and belt do you carry?

J: I like a nylon belt and front cross draw holster in the left position near the belly button. This along with a double magazine pouch made out of the same synthetic material.

STREET SURVIVAL LESSONS

1) *Target ID*. Be aware that drive-by killers may use stolen cars to throw you off guard.

2) *Disguises*. The use of disguises by drive-by killers in some areas of the world are making it even more difficult for would-be victims to react in time.

3) *Front, side, rear ambushes*. The techniques of handling front, side, or rear ambushes differ. Know how to handle each.

4) *The brake trick*. Applying your brakes just as a suspicious vehicle attempts to pass you may throw your would-be attacker off stride.

5) *Firing from right and left and front-side windows*. It is very important that a driver work out what gun rig and draw technique works best for him when having to cover the driver's- and passenger's-side windows.

6) *The side-swipe maneuver*. The use of an explosive counterattack by the side-swipe technique may save your life on the road. It is important to understand the disparity of size limitations of the

technique. An extreme example would be if your antagonist is in a trailer-truck and you are driving a small car. Such a disparity of force may cancel out the practicality of the technique.

WHEN DRIVE-BY SHOOTERS TARGET YOUR VEHICLE

If you have one or more armed passengers with you, you are in a much better situation than when you are driving alone. Never drive alone if you can avoid it, especially in ambush prone or isolated areas. An armed passenger can engage your enemy with more manual dexterity than you can, thus raising your street survival odds significantly.

Driver Plus One Armed Passenger

When driving with a friend, most people sit in front next to the driver. This is a tactical mistake. Drivers have great problems in traversing the handgun so that it can fire out the

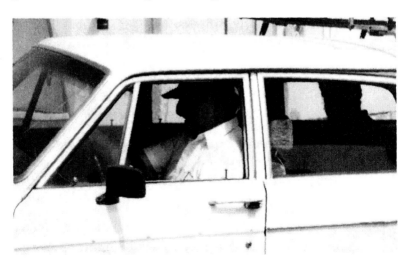

DRIVER PLUS ONE ARMED PASSENGER: An armed passenger sits in the shadows of the rear seat covering both open windows.

driver's window or the front passenger's window. Placing an armed passenger in the front seat does not really solve the problem since the passenger can only fire out of his window. A much more efficient thing to do, which increases the capability of successfully engaging an attack, is to place the armed passenger in the rear and have both windows open. The armed passenger can fire a short-barreled long gun or a handgun. To accomplish this best, it is imperative that the passenger sit in the middle of the rear seat. In doing this he is then able to cover both sides of the vehicle and, in a pinch, even shoot out the rear window and fire to the rear.

Driver Plus Two Armed Passengers
When having the good fortune of traveling with a second armed passenger, you would do well to place said passenger in the rear seat too. Have them each take a rear side window. Thus, each of the armed back-ups may then be able to handle attacks comfortably and in a most efficient manner.

I once thought of placing the second backup in front but now believe otherwise. I now recommend the rear seat to my students so that each back-up can fire out of the rear side windows, which offer better visibility and trajectory of fire than front side windows.

Driver Plus Three Armed Passengers
With a third armed passenger, the front seat next to the driver is the best place to be. In this case the backup can engage targets to the right while the driver can engage the much more easier (for him) targets to his immediate left.

Driver Plus Four Armed Passengers
A fourth armed passenger will sit in the middle of the rear seat and not be of much use unless the rear window is ejected or shot away. The need of having a rear window that ejects (also a good idea for the front one) is an idea whose time has come.

The VIP Vehicle
I have always been perplexed as to why VIP vehicles do

not have the capability of having their front or rear windows opened or even ejected in a firefight so that better traverse fire can be applied against an attacking enemy. Such a capability would enormously shift the odds back toward the intended VIP target in that for the first time a closed car would be capable of engaging targets in a 360-degree circle if the need arose—a very interesting and useful optional capability.

TRAINING: STATIC AND MOBILE MOCK-UPS

The best way to begin your practice is from a mock-up of the front end of a vehicle. A simple chair, a steering wheel held in your hand, and side "windows" cut out of carboard work quite well. Practice drawing your pistol, steering the car, and firing out of either of those windows. Of course, you will find that keeping your eyes on the road while engaging your target is impossible. This means you have to develop a workable solution. The thing to do is to turn your head, look out of a window, fire the instant you see the target, then snap back to look out of the front window. This can be done as needed, though unless you are being attacked by a vehicle driving alongside, you won't have time to do the maneuver more than once or twice since you should have raced past your attackers. Your armed back-ups fire from their positions with their own mock-ups. A bus company here uses an interesting idea. It has the driver sit at the wheel in a small vehicle that runs along mini-rail tracks. This simulates the problems one has to face when the bus is moving.

THE MOVING VEHICLE

Once you have mastered the techniques in the mock-up, you can go to your vehicle and train from it, engine on, as you gradually increase your speed with each turn at the wheel until you are functioning at road speed. This training technique is best done on a professional range under professional control of licensed instructors since safety precautions must be very stringent.

This is the ultimate way to train and can include not only the driver but armed passengers who will engage their targets as well. The use of realistic targets as well as so-called "innocent" targets, forcing you to think target selection, is a good idea with all training for firing at enemies who are ambushing you from roadside positions. The principles of safety, marksmanship, and target selection apply.

STREET SURVIVAL LESSONS

1) *Armed passengers.* Know how best to use armed passengers as backup when you are driving.

2) *Training behind the wheel.* Prior training is paramount to successfully carrying out survival scenarios on the road. This is done through the use of static or mobile mock-ups and, eventually, the moving vehicle. Good marksmanship, safety, and target selection are as valid and important as always.

WHEN PARKED OFF THE ROAD

There are times when circumstances may force us to park our vehicles in areas that we might want to avoid. When this occurs it is important to have worst-case scenarios planned so as to not be caught off guard.

Case History: How I Survived
Vehicle Breakdown in "Enemy Territory"

A few years back, I was in my military car when all four of its tires were blown out by hundreds of twisted nails strewn on the road in an Arab-populated town in Israel called Ramallah. We swerved to a sudden stop. My driver informed me that he would have to leave the car, flag down a passing army truck, and go back to base for four new tires.

As he looked around at the gathering crowd of about 50 onlookers, he informed me that we had one little problem. If we left the car unattended, we would return to a stripped and burnt-out hulk.

I told him to flag down the next passing army truck and I would baby-sit the car. Within 10 minutes he was gone and I was alone, except for those 50 onlookers.

I was next to a cafe that had some chairs and tables outside its entrance, but I decided to pass and pressed my back against the stone wall of the building, picking an area that even had a little extra protection, a piece of wall that jutted out about 6 inches so that my left side was further protected. It immediately became obvious to me that my fan club, who were eyeing my car and my anatomy, were somewhat taken aback by my maneuver. After a hurried meeting, they sent a smiling emissary toward me with arms spread wide, repeating, "Salaam, salaam" (Arabic for peace), all in a most friendly and disarming manner.

Imagine how disconcerted he was when I pointed down at a crack in the sidewalk and informed him that was the border; if he crossed it I would be forced to pump his anatomy full of lead. I repeated the message calmly and slowly. It was crystal clear. With this, he stopped in his tracks, turned to the crowd, and informed them of my most ungentlemanly statement. He then turned to me and invited me to sit outside the cafe in a chair that he placed in front of my car, its back to the expectant crowd. I coldly but politely reinformed him about that crack in the sidewalk. He stared at the .45 on my hip, then turned, throwing his hands up in dismay, and he and the disappointed crowd melted away.

What my hospitable emissary did not know was that I had my hand on another .45, a Colt LW Commander in a special, oversized jacket pocket that allowed a very fast draw. The gun's muzzle was covering him at all times.

An interesting thing occurred as I waited. An Israeli paratroop officer appeared seemingly from nowhere. He ran across the street to me, informing me that he had been driving up another street, had noticed the army car and some

Israeli standing against the wall with a crowd around him, and decided to check out the scene. He had been observing my behavior for a minute or two and decided to go on his way, but not before he decided I looked like I didn't need any help. He was right, my experience with King and the Israeli police had served me well. Like the Spartans at Thermopylae, I had allowed a potential enemy only one route of attack: directly at me. I proved to myself that when the rear and flanks were covered I could easily control the situation and, if need be, hold off a very numerically superior force.

Now all this may sound slightly paranoid, but I can assure you it is not. A few weeks later, an Israeli soldier was stabbed to death not more than a few hundred yards from where I stood. This was followed by an attack on an Israeli citizen with the same dire consequences.

I came to the firm conclusion many years ago that, given the choice, I would much rather be a nasty live paranoid than a very likable and trusting corpse.

STREET SURVIVAL LESSONS

1) *Don't forget back and side cover.* Use back and side cover whenever possible. The use of cover should not be restricted to frontal cover alone.

2) *You call the shots.* Never let a supposedly friendly street person place you in what common sense would call a compromised security position. Don't be afraid to be discourteous when your life is at stake. A number of Israelis would be alive today if they had acted in a discourteous manner and turned down rides offered to them by murderous rapists and terrorists. Common courtesy does not mean you have to be shammed into dangerous situations by criminals who know how to appeal to your better instincts. Let your survival instinct be dominant over your manners.

3) *Draw a red line.* Don't be afraid to confront someone you consider dangerous. I pointed out the consequences of crossing that crack in the pavement. It was my red line.

4) *Use subterfuge.* Trickery isn't always in the hands of street predators. You can use it too. While my potential enemies stared at the 1911 Government Model on my hip, I had them covered by the LW Commander in my oversized pocket.

....

Case Study: Call of Nature

Jonathan related to me the following recent story that somewhat resembles what happened to me in Ramallah when those tires burst. He says he used some of the lessons learned.

One morning I was driving alone in the "West Bank" on a very lonely road when I had to answer an urgent call of nature. I spotted an isolated and abandoned building up ahead. It looked run-down and deserted. I pulled in back, got out, and stood against the wall to urinate when a giant of a guy in a beard, dressed in the sort of white gown that fundamentalists wear, turned the corner of the building and made for me, smiling and saying, "*Salaam.*" I pulled my Glock 21 and told him in no uncertain terms not to come any closer. Israelis had been murdered in the area, and I was not about to be added to the list.

He pulled back in surprise and asked why I was pointing a gun. At this, he started to make for me again. I told him this was the last warning. He looked at me for a moment, smiled, then informed me of the fact that he considered me something special, adding that if all Israelis acted like me he wouldn't get an Islamic Fundamentalist Palestine. I told him he wouldn't get one anyway. At this he turned and walked away.

When I got to my pickup truck I noticed that my visitor

was joined by three other men dressed the same. They coldly stared at me as I drove off. Unfortunately, not being an officer of the law anymore and not having anything that would stand up in court, I drove away, quite frustrated but still very much alive.

Obviously, he and his cohorts had spotted me going behind the building alone and wearing a handgun that I am convinced they wanted very badly. Of course, his friendly act was a ruse to get close enough so that he could pull a knife, grab the handgun, and slice my throat in the process, or worse.

E.S.: Jonathan, what did you learn from this bizarre encounter?

J: To pee fast. Also, to pick locations when no proper and safe facilities exist that cast modesty aside and instead stress personal security. Pick open areas for pit stops, never an area that is easy for someone to approach without being seen.

E.S.: What about the vehicle?

J: I now park my vehicle like I did Stateside when I was in the police and making a felony stop. This means parking on the shoulder of the road with the front-end pointed at a 45-degree angle to the lane I just drove off. Then I crank the wheel hard to the left, exit, and move to the passenger side of the vehicle, standing at the front door post behind the engine.

E.S.: Why?

J: Drunks are attracted to lights, so if they ram the rear of the car at night or if someone deliberately tries to ram me in the day, the vehicle will spin around and stop them. I wouldn't be killed in the process.

I also like the idea of using the vehicle for protecting my left side, forcing an attacker on foot to come at me from the front or from the rear of the car at a 90-degree angle and where I'm ready for him.

E.S.: What distance do you feel comfortable with someone moving in on you?

J: As long as I am able to keep a would-be attacker at 8 yards or more and I am alert with gun ready, I feel I have a good chance of reacting fast enough to win. I try to use the engine, door posts, and tires as cover. Of course, rifle fire could get through some of that, but the engine does afford excellent protection against just about anything.

E.S.: I recently heard of a Russian immigrant woman waiting at a bus stop who was shot six times in the stomach in a drive-by shooting. Do you have any thoughts on how she could have used cover to avoid such an attack?

J: The principle is when you are standing at a semienclosed bus stop (Israeli design against bombs is concrete) or any such structure, do not go inside. It's better to stand at the edge of the front so that you can quickly react to threats coming at you from right or left. If the walls are thick, you may be able to use them as cover, an added benefit. A tree or telephone pole can be utilized in the same manner. I used to tell my police trainees before they went out on the street: "Tactics, tactics, tactics. Cover, cover, cover. Shot placement, shot placement, shot placement." In other words, know what is going on around you and think ahead.

Interesting enough, I received a phone call from the States from someone who had spoken to one of my former police trainees who wanted a message passed on to me.

It seems the officer had pulled over a vehicle with three men in it, and when they stepped out of the car, one of them pointed a gun at him. The officer felt that he was a dead man anyway, so he drew his weapon and triple-tapped 3 bullets into the perp's "10 ring." The perp never even got off a shot. Worst-case scenario training had resulted in tactics that paid off. The officer claimed that an explosive counterattack and good marksmanship had saved his life. He was right.

....

STREET SURVIVAL LESSONS

1) *Display your legal weapon or not?* There are two schools of thought as to the advisability of showing one's weapon if such action is legal: deterrence

(an armed potential victim may deter a would-be criminal) and attraction (an armed potential victim may draw an attacker who wants the weapon). Adapt each philosophy to your area of the globe. Jonathan was correct in showing his weapon, since he would have been a prime target for murder anyway.

2)   *Be wary of uncommon behavior.* Most men do not come close to other men when they are urinating, if at all possible. If this is true in the men's room, it goes double for field-expedient latrines. The mere fact that a male moved toward Jonathan when Jonathan was indisposed was a clear warning. This, coupled with the man's style of dress, was more than enough to put Jonathan on full-alert.

YOUR VEHICLE AS COVER

A passenger car, and, for that matter, almost all civilian vehicles, look more thick-skinned than they really are. Except for the chassis, axles, wheels, tires, struts for roof support, and the engine, most cars made today are about as formidable a barrier against even a pistol bullet as a can of warm beer. Therefore, knowing the inner anatomy of your vehicle is a prerequisite for using it for proper cover.

Field Test

Back in the early 1960s, I was doing research for a book I was writing entitled "The Complete Book of the .45 Auto." (I could not interest any publisher in the manuscript, being told that such a book would be of little interest to readers.) Talk about being premature. I'm sure such a book would generate some interest today, though the field may be somewhat saturated. At any rate, I spent a day in a junkyard firing .45 and 9mmP ball ammo at an assortment of junked 1940s and 1950s cars. This was when most American cars were still made with steel bodies that were thick and heavy.

I fired at wooden targets placed in the front and rear seats and was utterly amazed as to how easily both those calibers punctured the door and body and went on to zip through the target and sometimes smash against the engine, which, of course, stopped them cold. About the only obstacle in a door that acted as a barrier were the steel bars that moved the windows. Otherwise (unless the windows were down), those doors were perforated like Swiss cheese. (Consider how much more useless today's thin-skinned cars would be as cover against most handgun bullets, let alone rifles, shotguns, and submachine guns.) I saw enough to convince me that anyone foolish enough to rely on car doors and bodywork for cover would incur fatal wounds.

Which Calibers Work Best against Vehicles?

Almost all long guns will perforate today's vehicles with enough power to inflict injury on passengers, provided the barriers previously listed are not struck. Almost all handgun bullets, except for the so-called "mouse calibers," will penetrate as long as those bullets are of sufficient weight and velocity. This means loadings that are considered powerful enough for self-defense. Firing a light target load at a car is not what we are talking about in that you would not usually choose such a load for street carry.

Over the years, I have carried out many more tests on vehicles and have come to some conclusions. The velocity of a bullet is extremely important when hard barrier penetration is needed. We are not speaking of stopping power but rather penetrating power. All things being equal, when we compare velocity, bullet weight, and cross-sectional area (caliber), the speed of the bullet seems to be of utmost importance in breaching hard barriers. The higher the speed the better. The energy in foot-pounds is what we are speaking of.

There is a sharp gain in striking force with each incremental increase in velocity. This table demonstrates the dynamics of what occurs:

100-grain bullet
600 fps = 80 ft.-lbs.
850 fps = 160 ft.-lbs.
1,000 fps = 240 ft.-lbs.
1,200 fps = 319 ft.-lbs.
1,470 fps = 479 ft.-lbs.

Note that the energy increases quite rapidly as the velocity is increased, making for a marked increase in striking force. This ability to penetrate barriers can be a liability when engaging human targets, since the ability to overpenetrate a street punk and then go on to hit a baby in a carriage also increases. That is why carrying jacketed ball ammo, especially of the 9mmP variety, can be so dangerous on the street. Stick with hollow points that have a good chance for expansion if you want less dangerous results for innocent bystanders. A case comes to mind where such advice was ignored with almost fatal consequences to an innocent bystander.

Case History: Not Hardheaded Enough
The remnants of the Western Wall of the Second Temple (Herod's temple) are visited by thousands of tourists and worshippers every day. It was during a particularly crowded day that a woman terrorist decided to rush at a policeman, a knife in her hand. The Israeli officer pulled his Browning 9mmP and fired one shot, hitting the terrorist in the head. Unfortunately, the bullet used was 124-grain jacketed military ball, and it whizzed through the terrorist's head and went on to hit a pregnant woman. The shot seems to have been one that hit plenty of skull tissue and bone, but this did not stop the jacketed bullet from bringing down the innocent bystander, who was hit in the torso. Luckily, the innocent bystander and her baby lived. I can't say the same for the perp.
The public would have been better served if the officer had carried a hollowpoint cartridge in his Browning. The authorities should have issued the officer such ammo, since

he was on street and not on highway patrol. Keep ball ammo for car use if you want, though many of today's modern hollowpoints, such as those of 147-grain in 9mmP, do the job and are the choice for street and car use, expanding well in tissue and still having the needed option of metal and wood penetration. The sometimes falsely maligned 147-grain subsonic 9mmP is a good all-around choice (Black Talon has done well here) and cancels out the need for ball ammo unless one is on the military battlefield.

Overpenetration of Soft Targets

The problem of overpenetration is a difficult one that adds one more thing for officers of the law and civilians to worry about. This is not so much the case in the military, since most of the time anyone you are firing at is backed up by more enemies. On the battlefield, two for the price of one is very attractive.

For those officers and civilians carrying in the street, the problem of overpenetration can occur with any ammunition, and while it is something to think about, it must not interfere with the critical factor of taking out a criminal who is about to inflict deadly mayhem. The damage said criminal may do far outweighs the potential danger of properly selected ammunition overpenetrating to innocents.

"Spray and Pray"

There are new statistics that at first glance seem to make all of this fuss about overpenetration seem somewhat academic. The vast majority of shots fired at perpetrators by uniformed police and civilians wind up missing their intended target. This has been exacerbated by the carrying of all those high-capacity handguns, which tend to turn otherwise cautious former revolver men into "spray and pray" shooters. This said, there is no excuse for spray shooting, whether it be on foot or from a vehicle. Placing innocents in jeopardy by clouds of poorly aimed bullets or those that overpenetrate is to be avoided. The eternal rule is that there are no substitutes for good marksmanship and bullet selection.

Vehicle Penetration

We all know that as you increase the angle at which any bullet is fired against an object, the ability to penetrate is reduced markedly. You must keep this in mind when conducting any test. In testing, use the ideal frontal shot rather than shots very tangential to an object, since those type of angle shots usually vary too much to allow you to draw meaningful conclusions as to penetration. What you want are bullets that penetrate under ideal conditions so that you can choose them without being led astray by angle of flight.

Another factor in firing at vehicles is to remember that a pointed bullet is still the best shape for getting through car metal. Unfortunately, the same bullet is the least effective shape for manstopping chores. The good news is that many of the better hollowpoints actually close on meeting hard resistance and then penetrate like ball.

During testing, it has been found that expansion of a bullet does not necessarily stop penetration if you are pushing the bullet along with sufficient velocity. Many such hollowpoints will get through wood or metal barriers if they are pushed fast enough and have sufficient weight.

....

STREET SURVIVAL LESSONS

1) *Concealment isn't necessarily cover.* The engine, wheel wells, axle, and tires are the best cover you can find in a vehicle. In general, everything else looks like cover but in reality provides only concealment.

2) *Velocity.* All things being equal, bullet velocity seems most critical for penetrating hard barriers.

3) *Pointed bullets.* Pointed bullets penetrate hard barriers more efficiently that any other design.

4) *Know your bullet.* Know the effect of the car-

tridge you carry on soft and hard targets. Test what you carry. Chart its characteristics.

5) *Multiple-purpose hollowpoints.* With the fine variety of quality hollowpoint bullets available today, most with good feeding characteristics, one should select those examples that can be carried safely in urban areas so as to reduce the chances of overpenetration on soft targets while exhibiting the power to defeat hard targets when needed.

6) *Keep overpenetration in perspective.* Be conscious of the problem of overpenetration, but keep a sense of perspective. A killer about to gun down a crowd must be taken out.

....

Hitchhiker Madness

The cruel phenomenon of the brutal murder of hitchhikers and those picking up hitchhikers has made this once casual and socially acceptable practice questionable. In spite of this, hardly a day goes by that one does not see individuals hitchhiking. I've seen young girls get into cars whose drivers I would be hesitant to accept rides from. The deadly naiveté of many is most surprising.

Case Study: Hitchhiker Murders at Gush Katif

There are times when you may be tempted to accept rides from strangers, such as when your vehicle is broken down on the road, or when you need a ride and none is available at the time. The following is not a rare case of what can happen.

Not every enemy signals his intentions. Many times a ruse and camouflage are used to disguise evil intent. This is especially true when people insist on hitchhiking on the roads and highways of today. Both hitchhiker and Good Samaritan who picks him up have been used as subterfuge for murder. No better technique of setting unsuspecting people up for murder exists than in the persistent, sometimes deadly habit of hitchhiking.

Staff Sgt. Ehud Roth, 35, and Corporal Ilan Levy had just completed their yearly reserve duty stint in the Gaza Strip. The army told them that a group of Israeli settlements in the Strip called Gush Katif were located in a "safe area" an area from which it was safe to hitch a ride back home. That day, Roth and Levy were dropped off by a military jeep at the hitchhiking area, in the hope of finding a settler's car which would take them along the so-called eastern road and out of Gaza.

They did not have long to wait. A beige Subaru station wagon with Israeli license plates pulled up. The two "Israelis" in the front seat smiled, and the staff sergeant and corporal jumped into the back seat.

After a mile or so, the Subaru turned left toward Khan Yunis, a large town in the strip. A Hamas fundamentalist gunman then turned and shot the two soldiers with his pistol at point-blank range.

An Israeli colonel said the following: "There were signs of a severe struggle, indicated by dents in the inside of the car's roof made by the muzzles of the gun barrels of the soldiers' M16s."

The murderers took a shirt and both M16s, as well as both pairs of army boots and both of the murdered soldiers' ID cards.

The car was traced and found to have been stolen from Gan Yavne, an Israeli town. When the car was found, a leaflet was already being distributed in Khan Yunis that included a photo of Roth's ID card with his picture. The leaflet was distributed by the Ezzedin al-Kassam armed wing of Hamas, which took credit for the double murder. It said, "This is a gift of Hamas to the peace process. There is no peace between us and the Israelis except in the cemetery. The settling of accounts will continue until the day of judgment, as long as the trees say: 'Here is a Jew hiding. Kill him.'" (A phrase of Mohammed in the Koran, which appears in article 7 of the Hamas covenant.

STREET SURVIVAL LESSONS

1) *Do not hitchhike.* Picking up victims who need rides is a favorite ploy of criminals. Plan so as not to have to depend on rides from strangers.

2) *Do not pick up hitchhikers.* The reverse is true. Never pick up hitchhikers. Fake road accidents, pretty ladies on the road—all such ploys have been used to make someone stop. Be wary and cautious of such things. A criminal scam in Haifa, a large port city in Israel, was to have a pretty lady flag down a car for a ride and then have her boyfriend drive up and demand blackmail money or she would cry rape to the police.

3) *Beware of road trickery.* Dressing up as policemen, soldiers, clergy, etc. are tricks that are becoming increasingly popular with criminals on the lookout for victims. The same with the use of stolen vehicles and switched license plates. Some criminals are getting more tricky as the public's awareness of rising crime statistics increases.

4) *Rifles are not ideal in cars.* Probably no better example of the problem of having a long gun in a vehicle could be attested to than these horrible dent marks made on the murder car's roof as those two soldiers vainly struggled to bring their M16s into play as they were being murdered. (Had Roth and Levy had pistols on them that were ready for instant use, things might have gone differently.)

THE CIVILIAN CONVOY

Since road attacks are very difficult to defend against in

some areas of the globe, a convoy system of defense will give much added security. Firepower is obtained by increasing the number of vehicles and hence the number of armed individuals who can engage attackers. A gauntlet effect is created that deters would-be drive-by killers from attacking.

However, even in areas of the world where such defensive tactics are needed, they sometimes prove impractical, because ordinary people simply do not want to travel that way on a daily basis. Of course, we are not speaking of the military or special high-security cases such as VIP protection units, which have greater means of convoy protection at their disposal. We are referring to the problems of the average civilian who drives on roads dominated by criminals or terrorists. For these people, a special form of convoy system must be constructed, one that takes into account the limited resources of this group.

Case Study: The Hadassah Hospital Convoy Massacre

During Israel's War of Independence in 1948, a small Israeli enclave in the divided city existed on Mount Scopus where the Hadassah Hospital and the Hebrew University were located. The enclave was supplied by a convoy that passed through the Sheikh Jarrah Quarter, an area controlled by the Arabs. The British Colonial Forces were still in the country at the time, and they were supposed to keep the Palestinian Jews and Arabs apart, being responsible for the safety of the convoy. Unfortunately, this was not always the case, and in a short time the convoy was forced to become an armored one, protected by the Hagana, one of the three Jewish underground forces serving in Jerusalem.

Dr. Chaim Yassky, director of the Hadassah organization in Palestine, and his wife Fanny left on April 14 with heavy hearts, knowing that the enclave and hospital would have to be abandoned soon. New hospital facilities were being sought in the Jewish-controlled part of Jerusalem.

Esther Passman-Epstein, in charge of the hospital's social welfare services, had made up her mind to join the convoy. She wanted to pass around candy, magazines, and cigarettes to the few remaining patients there. She was shunted to one of two white armor-plated ambulances with red shields of David painted on them. These ambulances were soon joined by two armor-plated buses and three large trucks filled with equipment. Two armored escort cars made up the convoy. One would take up point and lead the convoy; the other would be the last vehicle in line. The armored cars, like all the other vehicles, were simply standard-type vehicles that had heavy boiler plate welded to them, making them unwieldy and difficult to control but reasonably immune to most rifle bullets.

When the steel shutters were all closed, a British police officer gave the all clear, and the convoy with 105 people moved off—the front armored escort car, Lassky's ambulance, the second ambulance, the two buses, the three trucks, and the rear escort car.

They drove along the road without any problems, and when they passed the mosque in Sheikh Jarrah everyone felt the worst was over. They were wrong. Just after they had passed a British army post at a turn in the road, the first escort car was smashed by an electrically fired land mine that spun it around. The driver of Yassky's ambulance slammed his brakes and the ambulance skidded, its rear wheels hopelessly mired in a deep ditch. Suddenly, all hell broke loose as Arabs hiding in ambush opened up with rifles, pistols, grenades, and Molotov cocktails. The sound of bullets clanging against boiler metal was deafening. Yassky took his wife's hand and whispered, "*Shalom* [good-bye], my dear. This is the end."

Behind the ill-fated Lassky ambulance, the second ambulance braked hard. Mrs. Passman-Epstein had been giving tea to one of the wounded on the floor and it spilled on a nurse who was nearby. The nurse screamed, "Oh my God! I'm bleeding!" When everyone realized it was tea they burst into laughter.

The ambulance driver tried to turn around, but as he peered at the narrow road through the slit, a bullet slammed into his face. A second driver took the wheel and, with great effort, succeeded in turning the ambulance and drove away at full speed, bullets clanging around him, saving them all.

The two large buses behind the second ambulance were much too unwieldy to turn around. They tried to advance, but the driver in the first bus couldn't see much through the thin slit in his windshield. Disaster struck as the bus slowly slid into the ditch. The driver of the second bus tried to move past and skidded into a ditch on the other side of the narrow road.

The driver of the second of the three heavy trucks wrenched the wheel and just avoided both ditches by looking through a tiny hole where a screw had fallen out of the steel plate on the side of his cabin.

His tires punctured flat by bullets, the driver's arms felt like lead as he wrestled with the wheel, turning the truck around. As he careened down the hill, his brakes went and he expertly maneuvered, arms numb, as steel wheel frames sliced through the smoking rubber tires. In his case, the swaying movement of the truck probably saved his life as the Arab snipers missed the slit in the armored plate he was squinting through. He was almost hit once by a bullet that squeezed through the slit from a most unexpected direction, the British army post. Such things did occur at that time. Individual British commanders and soldiers sometimes did such things, providing either Israeli or Arab with more than moral support, depending on which side they had sympathy for.

As the convoy continued receiving heavy fire, it could be seen that the first escort car was finished, the first ambulance and two trucks were stuck in ditches, and the rest of the vehicles were trapped on the narrow road.

The British authorities refused permission to the Hagana to mount a rescue attempt, saying this would torpedo negotiations they were having with the Arabs aimed at arranging a cease-fire. Realizing that the British would not intervene, the Hagana sent four armored cars, two from the city and two from Mt. Scopus, toward the site of the ambush. Heavy Arab fire forced them to retreat.

A lone, brave British officer in a partially armored car raced near one of the buses and shouted for them to come out and run across an open area to him. He knew they had a poor chance of making it, but he also knew they were doomed if they didn't try. His offer was refused. They thanked him, and the courageous officer drove away through a hail of fire.

The 13 passengers inside Yassky's ambulance had a growing feeling that they were all doomed as the fire directed at them grew into a storm. Dr. Yehuda Matot, a former British army officer himself, said he was going to make a run for it to try to get help. All agreed the attempt was suicidal, but he said he was going to try. He jumped out and moved up a hill raked by small arms fire. He was about halfway up the hill when he was hit in the back. He fell down, lying there for a moment, then began crawling ahead, slowly, painfully. Then he heard voices. He thought he was hallucinating when he spotted two British soldiers who were watching from the entrance of a house.

"Come on, come on, chum. Keep coming. Little bit more. You can make it," one of them called to him.

Matot summoned up his remaining strength and crawled through a stream of bullets that miraculously seemed to miss him. All the time, the curses of the Arabs could be heard above the din, and the voice of that British soldier: "Come on . . . come on." In what seemed an eternity, Matot inched forward and, as he started to pass out, he looked up and saw a British face, which smiled, "Blimey, he made it!"

The uneven battle churned on for hours. It was about 1 P.M. when Dr. Yassky spotted a British convoy drive past the area. In the convoy, General McMillan surveyed the battle and decided that he wasn't going to intervene militarily. Talking was less dangerous for himself and his men. Yassky moved back from the peephole and sighed his disappointment.

A second British military convoy came upon the scene. It also drove past the ambush, not stopping to help.

Meanwhile, from around the area, hundreds more Arabs were rushing to what looked like a great victory, adding to the noise and firepower that smashed against the trapped vehicles.

Meanwhile, from a casualty clearing station where the one escaping ambulance had taken her, Esther Passman-Epstein stood on the roof, viewing the battle. Then flames burst from one of the trapped buses, sending black smoke high into the sky.

"My God," she whispered. "They've set the buses on fire. They're burning them alive!"

The passengers in Yassky's ambulance heard frantic pounding on the door. A man yelled, "Get out, quick. They'll burn you alive!" A hail of bullets stopped the voice. Yassky peered out the peephole and saw the brave bus driver lying on the ground. "They've set the buses on fire," he gasped as he closed his eyes and died.

Arabs had set fire to the buses with Molotov cocktails, burning most of the passengers alive except for a few who had run from the door only to be cut to ribbons by a deluge of bullets.

Unknown to the passengers in Yassky's ambulance, the "peace negotiations" the British had pushed for had failed. As wisps of smoke filtered in, one of them had wanted to raise a white handkerchief as a sign of surrender, but the stench of the burning gasoline and the news of the massacre brought an end to any talk of surrender.

They calmly accepted the idea of their death. Better to be burned alive than fall into the hands of their tormentors.

An eery silence engulfed the inside of the trapped ambulance, in stark contrast to the screams, curses, and shooting that was whirling in through the tiny slits and peepholes.

Mrs. Yassky looked around the ambulance and felt that her husband was in an exposed position, sitting next to the driver, who also faced those slits from which the lead from the rifle bullets splattered in. He refused her request to move, saying that he would stay with the driver, who was in equal danger.

At about 2:30 P.M., Mrs. Yassky heard a groan and looked up to see her husband slump forward. She rushed to him. Blood was oozing from a hole in his side. She and the nurse tried to bandage him with bits of their clothing. She pleaded, "Darling, speak to me." Dr. Yassky didn't reply. A bullet had lodged in his liver, killing him instantly.

The others who had previously resisted running from the trapped ambulance now spoke of the attempt. What did they have to lose? Mrs. Yassky cradled her dead husband's head in her lap and looked up: "I won't leave my husband," she whispered.

Suddenly, Brigadier Jones, the local British commander, some six hours after he received the report of the ambush, ordered a heavily armed force accompanied by three military armored cars to open fire on the Arab positions. Within seconds, the superior firepower of the British caused havoc among the Arabs. Their attack against the convoy ceased.

Jones later claimed he needed the six hours to raise the force and that was why he hadn't intervened earlier.

Within a few minutes, the door of the trapped ambulance opened and a British major peered into the shadows. "I'm looking for Dr. Yassky and his wife."

"I'm Mrs. Yassky," she whispered. "This is my husband. He's dead."

The officer stared and then, in sympathy, whispered, "I'm sorry."

The Haddash massacre claimed the lives of 76 of the Jews trapped in the convoy, their burnt corpses including many top doctors of the Mideast. A pharmacist's body was missing, carried off by the Arabs as a trophy of war.

The Mt. Scopus enclave never was surrendered and was rejoined to the rest of the city when the victorious Israeli army swept past it in the 1967 Six Day War. A new hospital and campus now sit overlooking the panorama of the eternal city of Jerusalem.

The B-17 Convoy System

In designing a convoy that has to bring a number of civilian vehicles (the system also works in an emergency for the police and military) through an area where there is the possi-

bility of a well-planned ambush being carried out, I have recommended what I call the "B-17 Convoy System."

The idea is to view the convoy as a bomber flying through
enemy flak and fighter attack and to use the fire capability
that the World War II B-17 bomber possessed to survive. In
the system, the "nose" of the bomber could be an open pickup truck with an armed defender in the rear, protected by
sand bags and armed with a long weapon capable of laying
down a zone of fire to the front and side. This is followed by
"side gunners" (the vehicles that follow), who can protect
the convoy's immediate left and right. A second pickup can
be in the rear of the convoy to act as a "tail-gunner." If available, a third pickup truck can be placed in the center of the
convoy to act as a "top-turret" gunner. Increased cover
should be afforded these gunners in the form of light armor.

What is good about the B-17 system is that it is flexible in
concept, yet gives one a framework to build on. For example,
the pickup trucks can be increased in number or even replaced by larger trucks. The main idea is to place your firepower in a manner that is most effective against attack. (Of
course, in classic warfare, the military would protect flanks
of the convoy by mobile elements and air power would be
brought into play.)

Armor is critical, but it is kept in proportion and is not
stressed over mobility, vision, or effective firepower.

The use of mobile elements that can quickly debus is
another key element in surviving and then quickly turning
the tables on any ambushers.

As urban guerrilla warfare breaks out all around the
globe, fueled by economic unrest, the B-17 convoy system could prove a highly effective tool for laymen (and
police) who want to move a line of vehicles through a
riot-prone area.

I believe and trust in the merits of the B-17 system. It uses
the principles learned in flying unescorted bombers (flying
fortresses) over enemy territory. It incorporates the lessons
gleaned from the Hadassah convoy massacre. It provides a
useful framework for convoy survival.

STREET SURVIVAL LESSONS

1) *Convoy firepower.* Unless the firepower of a convoy can be brought to bear on an attacking enemy, the convoy simply becomes a line of ducks in a shooting gallery.

2) *Convoy visibility.* You can't hit what you can't see. Too much emphasis placed on armor at the expense of vision is wrong.

3) *Convoy maneuverability.* You cannot place more armor on a vehicle than its engine and chassis can manage. If the ratio of weight to power is exceeded, the vehicle becomes a coffin.

4) *B-17 convoy system.* Visualizing your convoy as a World War II B-17 bomber gives you a framework on which to build your fire-control system.

Chapter Eight

Securing Your Home from the Streets

*H*ere in Israel we use the three-circle defense system, a logical and orderly method of viewing your home defense problems. Each defense circle is constructed so as to discourage unlawful entry and slow down any violators of your home. The proper use of the three-circle defense system wins you and your family added and valuable time to arm and call for outside help. The three circles act as a layered defense system that is not only physical in construction but is mental in outlook. It is a logical way of viewing your environment in an orderly and structured manner.

The outer circle may be the outside entrance of your apartment building, the outer limits of your estate or home, or the outer limits of your village. The principles that go into constructing the outer circle are basically the same in all cases.

The middle circle consists of the actual walls, windows, and doors to your abode, your place of work, or any building for that matter.

The inner circle can be a safe room, an inner stronghold where a last-ditch defense can be mounted against an attacking enemy.

THE OUTER DEFENSE CIRCLE

Deterrence

You want the very look of the outer defense circle to quietly discourage unlawful entry, keeping in mind the simple fact that there is no way you can prevent an intruder from breaching any defensive barrier if he so desires. Even Fort Knox can be robbed. What you do want is to frighten or warn the culprit off and, if this doesn't work, to slow him down and then defeat him.

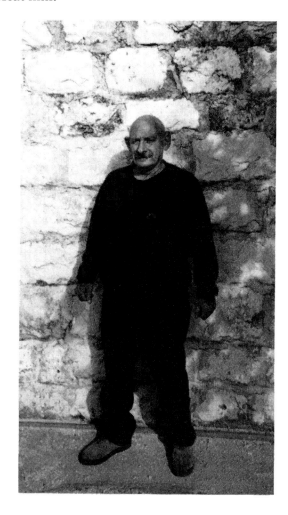

BAUM AT HIS OUTER DEFENSE CIRCLE: A stone wall.

Post Signs

Signs that proclaim the area as off-limits and dangerous to those seeking unlawful entry should be posted in plain view. Make these signs not only in the dominant language spoken but also in any second or even third languages that may be spoken in the area. Have the sign contain a picture that shows what the written part warns of. For example, a picture of a vicious dog is most unsettling to would-be trespassers and beats a lot of words on the subject.

The Fence

A fence can vary from a simple hedge, wooden pickets, wire, and stones to rolls of strung-out razor wire. In certain areas of the world, this can be augmented by such things as land mines and electric wire. Even a moat is something that works if you have the money and facilities to recreate such a barrier. The most important thing to keep in mind is that the outer circle of the area you want to protect must have distinct, well-demarcated boundaries. No one crossing such an area should be able to claim they had just wandered in. Have a locked door or gate with a nearby bell for those seeking lawful entry to press. Make sure the bell can be seen and easily reached from outside the perimeter defense. Don't give people bent on unlawful entry the excuse of saying they only wanted to ring the bell.

Barbed or razor wire is still the next best fence system to make life difficult for robbers or intruders. I said next best because the best system is the combination of electrical and barbed or razor wire that has sensors on it signaling not only that someone is attempting to enter your property but exactly where. Israel manufactures such fences, and they form the border between Israel and Lebanon. For civilian use, the problem with such a combination is that, besides the high cost, it is not aesthetic.

There is one other type of fence that could be constructed that has a "hot" high-current electrical wire on it. Such fences are out of bounds for use in democratic Western nations due to their lethal effects on anyone trying to breach them. The German SS used such fences around its concentration camps.

If you have the bucks, a brick or stone wall around your yard, topped by broken glass, spiked bars, or wire, makes an excellent outer circle fence. The problem with such a wall, however, is that it is very costly and out of reach for many. The same goes for most wire fences, though the cost of installation and material should be much less. Once again, such wire fences should be constructed so that it is difficult to climb over them. I remember scaling such fences with ease as a teenager when the school yard was locked and we wanted to play ball. Unless you add barbed wire to the top of such a fence, it poses no problem.

It is also a good idea to remember that not only can fences be dug under, but many can be breached by the use of simple wire cutters. Again, a fence can only deter or slow down someone who wants to breach it; it cannot be relied upon to stop someone from breaching our outer circle of defense. There is no barrier that can do that; not even the now-defunct Berlin Wall could.

Outer Landscaping

There is no logic in constructing a fence or wall demarcating your outer defense perimeter and then having tall trees growing nearby for people to climb over, thus defeating what you had built. True, we can have bushes act as an outer fence, but these should be thick and thorny enough for anyone to avoid like the plague.

All greenery should be cleared away from your fence or wall so that it does not provide a place to hide for anyone who got into your yard. Even the greenery that grows between the outer and middle defense circles should be pruned with an eye toward defeating its use as a place for anyone to hide behind.

Case Study: Kids Don't Obey Signs

Kids sometimes foolishly ignore clearly posted signs and even barbed-wire fences. I had such an experience a few

years back when a boy of about 10 who was visiting a neighbor decided to dig under the barbed-wire fence at the rear of
my farm and enter my yard. He wanted to pet a cute little
dog that I had. Unfortunately, he walked into another dog—
my Israeli Canani who was on a run that extended the length
of the back of my house. The Canani is a dog that appeared
in Biblical times and is noted for its warmth but also for its
fearlessness. Rex was his name, and he proceeded to mangle
the kid's leg with a series of very vicious bites.

The mother insisted I was wrong to have such a dog, and
the police were brought in to investigate. I showed them the
outer circle fence, which was well posted with signs. I pointed out the area the boy dug under. Rex was on a stout chain,
which held throughout the sorry episode. The boy had simply walked into his territory, and the dog reacted correctly.

An officer pulled me aside and informed me that the same
thing had happened to him a year back when someone came
into his yard. He was sympathetic to my claim that, unfortunately, the boy had done the wrong thing and in no way
could I or Rex be faulted.

The honest young boy came up to us and admitted he had
done a stupid thing. I felt sorry for him, since no one wants
to see kids hurt, but it wasn't my fault. It was his. Poor Rex
had to go to jail and be quarantined for a month, even
though I provided official papers that proved he had indeed
had his rabies shots. The case against me was dismissed.

Fence Lighting

One of the most critical additions in securing your outer
defense circle is proper lighting of your fence or wall and the
area between the outer and middle defense circles. A well-lit
area acts as a deterrence to would-be interlopers in that criminals do not relish working under spotlights.

There are two types of fence lights—those that go on at
night and stay on until dawn and those that are put on if you
suspect someone is in your yard. The best is to have a combination of the two. Then if someone tries to breach your
home, he may be warned off by those extra lights being

snapped on. Deterrence still remains the best policy, since what counts is getting a potential enemy to cease and desist, rather than having to engage him in a firefight.

....

STREET SURVIVAL LESSONS

1) *Three-circle defense system.* When constructing your home security system, think of it as being in three concentric circles.

2) *The outer defense circle.* This circle must show that you mean business. It must deter. To do this, clearly demarcate it by posted signs, fences, and good lighting.

....

THE MIDDLE DEFENSE CIRCLE

Outside Building Lights
The same lighting principles that apply to the outer defense circle (fence lights) go for the middle one as well. You cannot have enough lighting on your house or apartment. The lighting up of all dark and shadowy areas of your home's outer walls has a deterrent effect on prowlers.

Building Landscaping
Building landscaping must never provide needed cover for someone attempting to breach your middle circle of defense. Heavy bushes and trees next to the house not only provide a cloak for someone to work under, they can sometimes act as a ladder that can be used to climb up a building.

Keep all landscaping around your building low and not grown as full as you may like. Make it of no use to anyone attempting to get at you and your possessions. It makes absolutely no sense to spend money on good outside lighting and then conveniently provide dark areas for prowlers to hide in.

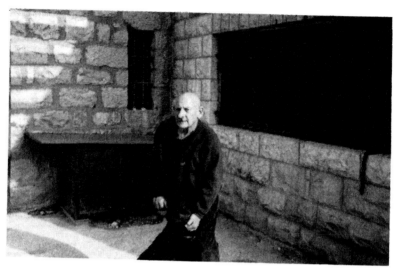

BAUM AT HIS MIDDLE DEFENSE CIRCLE: Notice the barred windows, lack of bushes, and Rottweiler dog.

Outer Door and Window Locks

Any lock devised by the brain of one man can be breached by the brain of another. "Burglar-proof" locks are a myth. That is not to say that some locks are not better than others, but all locks can be defeated by anyone given the time. The key word is time. Burglars are, by nature, nervous people who like to get in and out of a job fast. Complicated locks or groups of locks tend to take time to breach. They can act as another deterrent for our middle circle of defense. They also give us more time to respond.

I have wrought iron metal screen doors in front of the outer doors of my home. A friend of mine, upon viewing the doors, spotted a weakness. It was not in the locking system. I had enough of those. It was in the securing system that held the door to its frame. It then became obvious that someone wanting to gain entry only had to work on that portion of the door and could then bypass all its elaborate locks. So good locks alone may not do the trick. Check everything about the door if you want to slow up illegal entry of your premises.

Common Tumbler Lock

Most people have what is called the common tumbler lock. These work with a spring-loaded bolt system. When the door is closed, the bolt sits snugly in a recess cut into the door frame. The problem is that this type of lock has only one bolt, and once the bolt is disengaged, the door is easily swung open. These are the type of doors you see people in movies open with a plastic card slipped between the bolt and the door frame. Such a door has been "carded" or "slipped" for easy entry. You don't have to use a card, though. A knife blade or any thin piece of metal will do nicely. Burglars can do the trick in about 10 seconds. Avoid such locks like the plague.

Dead Bolts, Mortise Locks, Key-in-the-Knob
Locks with Trigger Bolts, Vertical-Bolt Auxiliary Locks

In the dead bolt design, the bolt is placed into the recess mechanically and so cannot be slipped or carded. However, a professional can still pick it and all of these locks with an easily obtainable set of lock picks and a crash course in picking locks gleaned out in the street or in prison. Some experts now believe the dead bolt design is really not the panacea it once was.

If picks aren't available, the old-fashioned skill called "jimmying" can be applied. This consists of prying or wedging a door open with a heavy metal bar. Some burglars here in Israel have upgraded the technique and use car jacks. After all, if car jacks can lift up a truck, they sure as hell have enough mechanical power to lift a door off its hinges. I've seen the results of such methods, and I can assure you, very few doors can withstand such applied mechanical leverage.

Windows (if unbarred) are no problem, since a suction cup with an attached cutter that is simply spun around in a perfect circle allows panes of glass to be lifted away noiselessly.

Alarm Push-Button Sequence Locks
and Keyless Binary-Coded Locks

These are the locks of the electronic age that are now on the market and in many homes. They can prove costly. Electronic gadgets now available to some burglars can circumvent the best of these, but at least they make him work for his money, and they take time to unscramble. These are definitely the locks of choice.

Inside Your Home: Locking all Inner Doors

When you leave your house, many experts suggest that it may be wise to lock all the inner doors. Since time is the enemy of the housebreaker, taking the time to open each and every door in order to check a room out works in your favor, not his.

Horizontal Cross Bars and Chains

If you are at home, the problem of securing doors and windows becomes much easier. Making your house as secure as a fort is best accomplished when you are inside the home. Heavy-duty safety chains on the doors in tandem with horizontal cross bars can make for very stout defenses. Some of these bars have now been upgraded to have a horizontal bar-lock and a floor-to-door bar-lock combo that is impervious to everything but an Abrams tank, or at least sledgehammers swung by Attila the Hun and his gang.

Case Study: Beds Aren't Always for Sleeping

Bruce, an immigrant from the United States, now lives out in Tekoa, an isolated Israeli settlement. When one of the residents of Tekoa was gunned down on a lonely stretch of road leading to the settlement, a widespread manhunt was mounted by security forces. They got their man, just as they eventually do with most of the murderers who carry out such crimes. He turned out to be a resident of an Arab village that could be seen from Bruce's dining room window. (He pointed it out to me as we were eating.) Bruce asked me for technical advice on how he could increase security in his home. He was upset that his son had taken to sleeping with a Boy Scout knife tied to a long stick. I shared some ideas and principles with him. Being on a tight budget, he knew he had to come up with some low-cost answers.

A few weeks later, Bruce told me the Boy Scout knife had

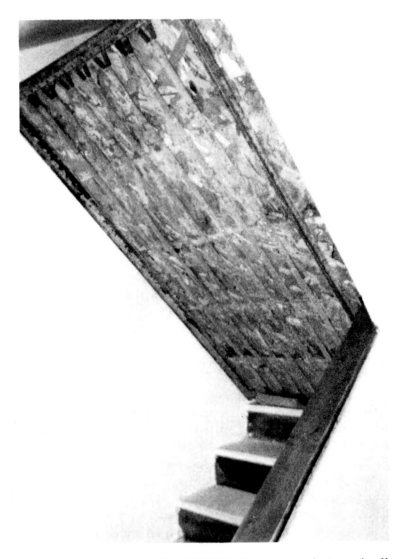

BRUCE'S LOW-COST BED BARRIER: This ingenius device seals off the top of the stairs leading to the second floor of his home.

been put aside because of something he had installed at the top of the stairs leading to the upstairs bedrooms. We went upstairs, and it turned out to be the metal framework of a bed minus the legs.

This he planned to strengthen and cover with wood. The whole apparatus was hinged so that it was raised during the day and then lowered and secured during the night, effectively cutting off the downstairs of the house from the second floor.

Bruce had also added an interesting touch, a few firing ports in the concrete wall across from it that allowed him to fire down at anyone attempting to breach the obstacle he had so cleverly designed.

What is important about the idea is its simplicity and very low cost. (NBC News thought it interesting enough to film it all for U.S. television.) Bruce's simple bed-spring barrier proves that not every solution to a home security problem has to be elaborate or costly. His was a practical solution to a very real threat. He is now in the process of carrying it out in combination with other ideas that will give him and his family improved chances of survival.

Metal Bars and Screens

The use of metal bars to slow down illegal entry is very widespread in the Mideast and southern Europe. The reason may be that most buildings are made of some sort of stone, so the threat of fire and being trapped inside of them is reduced. However bars and heavy metal screens can be placed on windows even in wooden structures if they are on hinged frames that can be locked or swung open. I am a believer in metal window bars and metal bar doors as secondary doors and have them on all windows and entrances to my home. And when I say all, I mean just that. Thieves bent on gaining entry will spot even the smallest opening.

We have a small food store in our village whose owner learned this fact the hard way. He placed metal bars on all windows except for a very narrow and tiny one that was near the roof of the building. When he went to open the store one morning, he looked up to see that the window was broken open and that the store had been robbed. It seems the robbers had used a child to accomplish the task; his small size found the window to be no serious barrier to entry.

Metal bars and screens can look very formidable, but once again they are only used to deter or gain time for the homeowner to suitably arm himself. Hack saws and crowbars can easily defeat these items, as can a chisel and hammer that chips away at their supporting structures. Even if the bars are made from hardened steel, a blowtorch will cut through them like butter. They are there to gain you time. A determined opponent will eventually breach them

---

STREET SURVIVAL LESSONS

1) *The middle defense circle.* Once again, proper lighting is critical along with well-trimmed landscaping that provides no cover for those bent on illegal entry into your building.

2) *Properly designed outside doors and windows.* Outside doors and windows should have proper locks, metal bars, or screening. Metal window bars can be hinged to metal frames so that the danger of being trapped in a fire is eliminated.

3) *Correct locks.* There are many types of locks in use. Use only the best ones for serious home security needs. Know which ones they are.

4) *Lock all inner doors.* When you leave home, it is prudent to lock all inner doors as well as your outer doors. Anything that slows up a criminal is to your benefit.

5) *Extra heavy-duty protection.* When you are at home, it is very easy to secure your doors with

heavy-duty safety chains in tandem with horizontal crossbars. Horizontal bar locks and door-to-floor bar-lock combos also work extremely well.

6) *Security doesn't have to be expensive.* Even an old bed spring can be used to block a hallway from illegal entry.

7) *Fire-ports.* The use of fire-ports that allow one to fire upon intruders is not a new idea. They were used to good effect by the defenders of castles centuries ago.

THE INNER DEFENSE CIRCLE (SAFE ROOM)

Another name for the inner defense circle is the so-called safe room. This room fulfills the role that a second, smaller inner castle did when men lived in castles. Every castle worth its salt had such an inner castle that was the area for last-ditch defense. This was a building constructed so that the few could hold off the many. That is the principle behind the modern safe room.

The inner defense circle, enshrined in the concept of the safe room, should be a well-planned and thought-out enterprise. It is the heart of your family's defense against the street.

Communications

A critical component of a successful safe room is having good communications capability in it. Simply being in the safe room is not enough to ensure your family's long-term survival. The safe room is only another means of buying you precious time until the authorities arrive. In time, even if properly constructed, defenses can be breached by a determined enemy.

Today, it is possible to have excellent low-cost communications from your safe room to anywhere on earth—certainly to your local police station. Of course, phones should be placed around the home, distributed with an eye toward security. Extension phones are a must. But the one or ones in the safe room are your real insurance policy. Certainly one phone should be of a wireless design so that it can't have its wires cut from outside the safe room. A walkie-talkie is another good idea. The main thing is that you are not dependent on power lines that can go out in a storm or be cut by criminals. You are independent of the outside, hopefully for enough time for help to arrive.

Loudspeaker
Another good idea I have set up in my safe room is a loudspeaker system. Imagine blasting out a warning for the whole neighborhood to hear when someone is trying to knock down the door of your safe room. It's certainly a novel way to use sound as a psychological weapon and alert your neighbors.

Siren and Revolving Light
Another idea is the use of a siren in the home with a revolving light. The whole apparatus can be set up on your roof or outside your safe room window. Hanon had a large siren on the roof of his house.

Anyone trying to get at you and your family is going to be nervous, afraid of detection, worried about the police arriving on the scene. A psychological warfare item such as the siren with blinking light can throw an enemy off balance as well as let others know you are in trouble.

Inner Circle Doors and Windows
The door to your safe room should be constructed of very stout materials that will withstand a series of very heavy blows directed against it. The door to my room is made of metal and has a four-way bar system securing it to its metal frame. For aesthetics, a veneer that resembles light walnut wood takes away the look of cold metal.

Since the room is on the second floor, it should be easier to defend against forced entry. Windows sport wrought iron

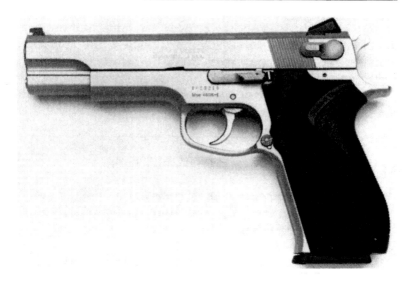

S&W MODEL 4506-1: An excellent handgun in .45 ACP for home protection. The magazine disconnector renders the loaded gun safe when the magazine is out. However, be forewarned that kids find everything that is hidden. Merely hiding a loaded magazine is not enough for home safety.

bars. A heavy elastic roll-down screen insures added privacy and security. It can be locked. I am thinking of having it replaced by one made of metal.

Inner Circle Weapons

Weapons and ammunition should be stored in the safe room. It makes no sense to keep your weapons and ammunition outside the safe room when you plan to use it as a sanctuary and last-ditch defense stronghold. By having your weapons and ammunition outside the safe room, you may inadvertently arm your enemy.

I had a good friend named Norman who used to hide pistols in nooks and crannies around his apartment in case someone broke in and he couldn't get to his guns. He was particularly partial to Luger pistols. While the practice worked nicely for him, it had serious flaws. Even though he had no children around, the system still lent itself to accidents by curious visitors. And it still meant that someone who broke into his apartment could find a loaded weapon. Better construct a proper middle defense circle that allows you time to retreat to your safe room rather than rely on such tricks, which could backfire on you.

STREET SURVIVAL LESSONS

1) *Inner defense circle (safe room).* There really can be no security for you or your family unless you have a proper safe room to retreat to when needed.

2) *Independent communications.* The safe room should have communications that are independent of any outside power lines. You must be able to communicate with the outside world.

3) *Psychological warfare.* The use of a loudspeaker system and/or a siren with lights is a good form of psychological warfare that not only has an unsettling effect on an enemy but can signal to others that you are under attack.

4) *Security door and windows.* The door and windows of a safe room must be secure from immediate forceful entry. A security door and barred or heavy screened windows are necessary to win you more than enough time to call for help. Arm yourself, and then react with lethal force if needed.

5) *Guns in safe room.* If a master bedroom is used as the safe room, it is the best place to store guns and ammunition. Never leave guns around the house. You may arm an enemy or have an accident.

BURGLAR ALARMS

Once upon a time, home alarm systems were very expensive, used only by the wealthy. Things have certainly changed. A mass market spurred on by an alarming increase in street crime has made home alarms as common as dishwashers. Some units are so simple a homeowner can install them himself simply by following instructions. This is a big money-saver and brings such systems to everyone. And because of a growing market, we have a better selection of alarms to choose from.

Home alarms are part of the middle defense circle, though they can be a very important element of the outer circle as well. There are four types of alarms in general use that come to mind for home needs. Each system has its own particular strengths and weaknesses, including cost of installation.

Electric Eye Alarm

The electric eye home alarm depends on photoelectric sensors to detect the presence of an intruder. It works by the simple system of a constant light being beamed to a sensitive photoelectric cell. If an intruder walks past the beam, momentarily cutting it, a sensor activates an alarm. The system works very well in guarding hallways, hatchways, and doorways. The problem is that to completely cover your home you would need dozens of sensors, strategically placed and camouflaged. Another drawback is that the system probably needs a professional to install it properly, thus adding to the cost.

Conductive Tape Alarm

This alarm system uses a network of conductive tape through which electricity constantly flows. The tape can be placed on all entrance points in the house, such as doors and windows. If the glass of a window that has this tape is broken, the tape will go with it and the electrical circuit will break, thus triggering the alarm. Some people like to have the alarm system trigger a buzzer in the police station or in a security office. The system can range from moderately priced in its simplest form to costly in its more complicated design. All depends on how elaborate you want it.

Ultrasound Alarm

This is a very advanced system that depends on inaudible sound waves that move out in a cone-shaped pattern. It can be adjusted so that it is triggered when a human being moves within the field of sound. If this occurs, the reflected sound waves bounce back to the unit and set off the alarm. What's nice about the system is that it can be made quite small and very portable, allowing it to be hidden in almost any reasonable-sized object in the room.

Some designs can be battery operated and or plugged into a wall socket. The system can be connected so that it closes gates, windows, etc., and turns on lights as well. Being moderately priced puts it into the range of most homeowners. You may only need one unit if you can figure out the best place to place it. It can be used both in the middle defense circle or as a vital component of the outer defense circle. This is a good system.

Circuit Breaker Alarm

The circuit breaker system is made to cover all entry points in the outer or middle circle. It is a low-cost system made up of small magnetic contacts that are connected by wires to a battery-operated alarm. The contacts can be attached to windows and doors throughout the house or to an outside gate. If a door, gate, or window is opened, the circuit will be broken, thus triggering the alarm or a bell, putting on lights, etc. A nice feature is that the central control box which controls the system can be set for "at home" or "away from home," so the inhabitants do not set off the alarm inadvertently. A manual operation alarm button is optional. The system's reliable, inexpensive, and can be installed by homeowners. This is a very good setup.

SECURITY DOGS

In areas where it is feasible, a good dog (or dogs) is a very important addition to keeping the street out of your home. Dogs can be trained to guard, attack, or just bark. The main thing is to have your dog properly trained. Leaving it all to chance is not the way to go. We recently had some terrorists murder a lone tractor driver who lived in a trailer on someone's farm. As the police carried out his mutilated body, I noticed two very forlorn dogs chained to the trailer. It seems they did not perform as their now deceased master had hoped.

We must keep in mind that dogs have rather distinct personalities, just as humans do. Some are fighters, others are lovers. Some are even both. Not all canines are defenders of territory. Not all canines will defend their masters instinctively if they sense danger. Some dogs will do both. If you have one that has a dual personality, consider yourself lucky.

Should You Train Your Dog?

Almost any large, strong dog can be trained for guarding the outside defense circle by being on a chain, run, or just roaming. This can be done by you or by a professional dog trainer. Most dogs begin their serious training at about four months of age, but this can be preceded by treating the puppy in a manner that encourages his natural aggressive tendencies. Do this by playing, fighting, and wrestling with him in a rough-and-tumble way, being careful not to injure him, of course. There are many excellent books on the subject that feature obedience training by voice command and demonstration.

Some training programs make the dog suspicious of all strangers. For example, a friend can act the part of the unwelcome stranger the dog attacks on command. This takes a brave friend who agrees to wear protective clothing. Teaching the dog to bite if you are attacked and to respond to voice control is serious business and takes lots of savvy, patience, and know-how by the owner.

Personally, I do not like or recommend do-it-yourself dog training, since a "failed product" could be very dangerous to everyone concerned, including family and friends. I much prefer and recommend that the professional dog trainer do the job if the goal is producing a biter who is a vicious attack dog.

Type #1: The Barker

If you desire a dog that is a living alarm system, the barker is the dog for you. Barkers can be used to guard the inside of your home or be on an outside chain, run, or allowed to roam freely. Such an animal is a mobile alarm system and can be any size or shape since you are not asking the animal to attack an intruder, just to bark at him. However, an added bonus would be to have the barker be a large, vicious-looking animal. Then his bark, while still definitely worse than his bite, would make people even more nervous.

Any dog may warn you by barking if someone enters "his" area, since most dogs are territorial by instinct and will usually bark if a stranger turns up. But you can't always count on that. You may have an erratic animal that may decide not to bark and will instead welcome an intruder or hide under the bed in utter silence. So even with the loud barker, proper training is the key to performance.

Type #2: The Biter

The biter will come to the defense of human beings and the property of human beings, namely his master. Such a dog means you have to spend time and money cultivating these traits so that you have an animal that performs 100 percent of the time. This is a responsibility not only for the dog but for its master. When a dog is a biter, you had better have a trained biter and not a loose cannon. Some dogs, when excited, strike out at any target within their chained area. I've actually seen some dogs bite themselves when they could not get at a human target.

Type #3: The Area Guard Dog

An area guard dog is a dog that has been trained to guard and patrol a specific area, in this case, the outer defense circle. The area guard dog is one that is trained to run loose in a well-fenced-in area. Such a dog can be a problem because he is basically on his own, roams freely, and will attack anything that enters his area of the circle. This is a canine that has been professionally trained to attack and neutralize any intruder without mercy. Such a canine is a four-legged lethal weapon whose one aim in life is to have someone enter his guarded perimeter so that he can perform the task he has been programmed for. Such a dog considers everyone but his owner fair game.

Now that we have described the area guard dog, it is obvious that such a creature must be contained behind very strong and high fences. This is an aggressive, vicious animal who is absolutely fearless in the attack. Many experts feel that such an animal should never be considered a family pet and do not recommend such an animal for the average homeowner.

This is an animal that is best suited for the large private estate, factory, or military installation surrounded by high walls. Here the area guard dog is taught to accept all members of the family, workers, or security personnel. Have such training done only by a professional who knows what it is all about, or you may face the danger of such a dog tearing apart a "friendly."

Anyone purchasing such an animal and wanting him as a house dog would be making a monumental error. By training, this dog is taught only minimal obedience, since in theory the trainer wants him to keep his most primitive instincts and mannerisms. He doesn't want to civilize the animal, only control him. If you have the facilities, such an animal is the best living burglar alarm ever invented, and he knows it. This is an animal not recommended for the average home owner.

Type #4: The Command Attack Dog

Any attack dog must be considered extremely dangerous, even one that is trained to attack only on command. If ordered to, such a beast will attack and rip apart any target. This creature is extremely fearless. Even wounded, he will continue with his task of neutralizing any threat with his dying breath. He is every bit as deadly a weapon as a crossbow or gun, and by law, you the owner will be held account-able for his actions, just as if you squeezed a trigger.

There is one thing, however, that makes the command attack dog somewhat superior to a crossbow or gun. He can be recalled and placed on guard once he has neutralized an enemy. It must also be understood that a very good thing about such a creature is the fact that if well trained, he will not attack anything unless ordered to do so by his master. Here is a dog that is a pillar of self-control and discipline. He is potentially very dangerous, but his training may make him actually safer to have around the family than a common house dog since he will take a certain amount of abuse with-out losing his cool. That is why he is the dog police select for use in riot control. In such work, the command attack dog is still usually kept leashed.

There may be times when the command attack dog func-tions without command and utterly and mercilessly neutral-izes an enemy. For instance, if his master is attacked and hasn't had the opportunity to call out the attack command, the dog should still respond without hesitation, tearing his target to pieces with jaws that exert more than 750 pounds of pressure and are lined with huge, sharp fangs.

These dogs are costly, sometimes running a few thousand dollars apiece, since their basic training takes time—as long as three to four months. This training means that not only the dog but you must be present, since the professional train-er wants the dog to bond to your voice commands. However, once you and the dog have graduated, you both must return for refresher courses on a regular basis.

Clearly, the acquisition of such an animal is costly and time-consuming and must be undertaken only by very seri-ous dog owners interested in street survival. Many experts caution anyone against purchasing such a dog already trained and bonded to someone else, since even with serious retraining you might never totally have a dog that has a 100-percent bond to you and you alone.

The good thing about such command attack dogs is that they, unlike the area guard dog, can be a family pet—a dog that can live in your home or take a stroll down the street with you. Such a dog should be safe with the elderly or with children, though I personally do not like any animal to be left alone with infants or toddlers. (I've read too many cases of German shepherds chewing off the fingers of infants, in spite of the fact that experts trust such animals under all circumstances.)

Another problem that can arise is when you find yourself away from home and the dog is alone with your family. Once again, training, is the key. If you are in such a situation, it may be best for your family to be bonded to the dog during his training so that he responds to their voice commands as well as yours. It is important to remember that all this takes work and love as well as a lot of patience. The responsibility is enormous when you have such an animal, but if the bonding is correct and the training done by a professional, the combination is hard to beat.

A few years ago, I spoke to someone who had used such highly trained command attack dogs in special operations that will remain unnamed. He informed me they could easily leap over a series of high fences, rip the Adam's apple out of an enemy guard's throat, and leap back to their trainer within seconds, all in complete silence. The guards never knew what hit them. These were undoubtedly the kings of command attack dogs.

Case Study: Fangs Galore

A few years back I had quite a slew of dogs around the farm, eight in all. All were barkers, and of these, five were biters. I kept them on chains placed in strategic locations that covered any approach to my house. No one could approach my house without having the gross misfortune of bumping into one of these canine alarms. Now one may rightly ask, why eight dogs? The answer is my younger daughter, Debbie, who was at home at the time, never let any dog go hungry. There were lots of hungry dogs around.

Their value was put to the test when the police chased two car thieves into our little settlement. The two perpetrators jumped out of their stolen car and made a beeline for my farm—this at 3 A.M. What they ran into was a canine nightmare. As they tried to cross the farm, each path they took was covered by a vicious dog on a chain. The perps ran around in circles as flashing fangs came out of the night and struck at them, all of this against a chorus of loud barking by my trained dogs.

In a panic, the perps ran back to the police and gladly gave themselves up, wanting nothing more to do with such a place.

The local police and my neighbors still cackle when they recall the story of the night of the fangs. For me, it was an excellent test bed of the validity of the use of multiple dogs for home security. Its effectiveness exceeded any expectations, except for one problem: who can afford to feed eight dogs?

NO ONE AT HOME?

Making it seem as if someone is at home when the house is actually empty is a good way of deterring break-ins. These following are some useful ideas that can fool burglars.

Barking Dog Tape

I did get an additional valuable idea from the experience—the use of a tape recorder of a barking dog in the house for when the house is, in fact, empty. The tape can be preset to go off if anyone rings the doorbell or tries to touch a window or door.

Time Clock

Time clocks are very popular in these parts, being used to put lights on and off for the Sabbath. The timers can be adapted to turning lights on at preset times when the owner is not at home. They are also very useful in putting on a radio. I usually pick a station that airs lots of talk shows so that human voices can be heard coming from somewhere inside the house.

One error not to make is leaving your front or back door lights on when the sun has not yet set. This is a tip-off to burglars that chances are no one is home.

Another thing to avoid is the accumulation of mail, newspapers, etc. at your door. It doesn't take a genius to see the house is empty.

Never place something in the local newspaper that informs the public of the fact that you will not be at home. For example: The Joneses have just won a free trip to Bermuda. Always try to enter the thought process of someone wanting to breach your middle defense circle. Anticipate things before they happen and you may just avoid problems.

Blinds Drawn
I make it an ironclad rule to close the blinds on all windows when the sun goes down. Never place yourself in the tactically incorrect position where people can see you and you can't see them. It's amazing how many people have no idea of this, feeling that if they can't see anyone, they can't be seen.

We have had the misfortune of people being shot through such windows by killers who capitalized on the situation of seeing their victim while they themselves were out of sight.

Case Study: Heights of Foolishness
We had a recent case of a young woman learning the hard way that living on the third floor of an apartment house offers no safety to a determined rapist.

It was one of those hot, humid summer nights in Tel Aviv, a large city on the Mediterranean coast of Israel. Donna had just gotten back from work in the wee hours of the morning, and she flopped down on her bed, naked, trying to get some of the little gusts of wind that came up off of the ocean. She left her window wide open; after all, she was on the third floor.

Now, Donna should have known better, since the case of a rapist who specialized in climbing up balconies to attack women had been well covered on TV for many weeks. So far he had eluded capture.

She closed her eyes and started to doze off when she heard something bang against her balcony. She looked up to see a man running at her. He jumped on her and they struggled on the bed. As they did, she managed to reach down and grab a .25 auto from a small holster she kept hanging from the side of the mattress and fired a single shot into his chest. He fell back, dead.

At the inquest, the family of the rapist screamed that she was a murderess who had killed their kin. They threatened to get even. The police warned them otherwise. Donna now closes her windows at night and has installed air-conditioning.

While the handgun saved her from being raped, it is not recommended that loaded guns be kept at bedside. There are cases where individuals, woken from a deep sleep, have mid-handled firearms that were close at hand in a state of panic. Better to have a properly secured home that provides some warning of someone breaching its defenses. This provides one with enough time to wake up and respond with all mental faculties functioning properly.

ID Chart for Valuables

It is wise and prudent to have a list of valuables that you keep in the home so as to assist the police in the eventuality that your home is robbed.

ARTICLE	MANUFACTURER	SERIAL NUMBER	SPECIAL MARKINGS
Camera	_____	_____	_____
Video	_____	_____	_____

For art, antiques, and jewelry, have a list that describes the type of material, shape, size, and mode of use.

....

STREET SURVIVAL LESSONS

1) *Four types of home burglar alarms.* There are roughly four basic categories of home burglar alarms. Know which one suits your particular needs.

2)   *Four types of home security dogs.* Know the four
      types of home security dogs. Know which type of
      dog best fills your needs. A professionally trained
      dog is more reliable than just any dog.

3)   *No one at home.* When you leave home, consider a
      barking dog tape and a time clock to turn lights
      and radios on and off. Never allow newspapers and
      mail to accumulate on your doorstep. Cancel the
      newspaper and have the post office hold your mail.
      Never announce that you are away from home.

4)   *Blinds drawn.* At sunset, draw all blinds so that
      no one can see into your home.

5)   *Height isn't safety.* Never believe that living above
      the first floor immunizes you from forced entry.

6)   *ID chart for valuables.* Having an ID chart for
      your valuables helps the police help you. A sepa-
      rate list for art, antiques, and jewelry is a must.

WEAPONRY FOR THE HOME

In some places in this world, home weaponry laws are far
more lenient than those pertaining to street carry. If you live
in a place that only allows you a house firearm, buy one.
Knives, clubs, karate, and frying pans aside, you can't beat a
hunk of lead traveling at high speed to make a perp cease and
desist. Only rely on "cold" weapons when you have no
choice and are not allowed a firearm. However, if you cannot
obtain a firearms permit, I most emphatically suggest you
obtain a long, razor-sharp sword. As I have previously stated, the sword is a superb, too-long-forgotten weapon ideally
suited for the home.

Firearms Safety in the Home

Hiding a firearm from a child may be a formula for grief. Kids just seem to find anything you hide and sometimes can even get by the elaborate security precautions you have taken. When my children were small, I made it a point to show them my guns. They were told they could fire them under my strict supervision, but they were never to touch them without my express permission, since they were very dangerous. They were especially not to allow their friends to see or touch them. My son fired a Colt .45 auto at the age of 5 and was quite satisfied about the contract I made with him. He kept to the bargain until his adulthood.

This contract worked for my family. It may not work for yours. All parents have to make an evaluation of their own children. Some may want to have firearms locked up at all times. Very good security boxes are being sold for this express purpose. Just be careful about the key falling into someone's hands. My daughter took my advice and hangs the key around her neck. She is not happy about the idea but is even more unhappy about the idea of it falling into the children's hands.

The American National Rifle Association has literature on the subject of home firearms safety. It may be wise to read it and carefully evaluate your particular home firearm safety needs.

HOME TACTICS AND TRAINING

All the passive defenses around your home have been developed with one thing in mind—helping you gain time so you can handle a breach of your middle defense circle. The inner defense circle is the place to retreat to if you have such a place and the opportunity to lock a security door behind you. Don't be a hero and go hunting through your home for armed intruders unless you know what it's all about. You must be very familiar with MOUT (Military Operations in Urban Terrain) techniques and have a good understanding of police reaction patterns (you don't want to shoot or be shot by responding police officers).

The First Priority

Anyone who faces the important task of protecting his family must develop a sense and appreciation of priorities. Protecting the innocent is the real duty of the head of the family. You must secure the defense of the innocent before you even think about engaging a street predator, unless, of course, he is upon you. Take your charges to the safety of the inner circle defense room. Put them behind cover in your well-stocked and prepared "fort." Once they are all protected, you can turn to the task of handling the intruder in a much calmer manner.

Which Room Is Safe?

In picking your inner circle defense room (safe room), you have to take certain problems into consideration. First, the most vulnerable time of the day is in the evening when you and your family are asleep. That is why the master bedroom is usually chosen as the safe room. Unfortunately, many home designs put this room at the end of a hallway after the children's bedrooms. This is all wrong from a home security standpoint. The master bedroom should be in front of the children's bedrooms and command areas of entry.

The Single Parent Safe Room

For single parents living alone with the kids, it may be a good idea to use a child's bedroom as the safe room. Having to arouse and move sleepy small children at night in an emergency situation may prove difficult. It may be much easier to go to them and simply lock their security door behind you.

If you have such a situation, you should, of course, still store any firearm with you in your bedroom until it is needed and you go to the safe room.

The Family Works as a Team

If you have a spouse and children that are responsible and grown-up enough to use firearms, you have a very good defensive situation and a much superior inner circle defense. Such a team can practice emergency drill procedures so that each member of the family has a specific assigned task. For example, the wife can act as the communications officer, staying on the phone with the police and covering the door of the safe room with a firearm in hand. The older child can guard the window against ambush.

What you decide upon is dependent on the design of the room and the numbers and maturity of the children.

Some scenarios have the husband covering the access point of the approach to the safe room in what is called an interdiction position, such as is done by the military. The husband then moves into the safe room when all the family is ensconced in it. Such a procedure, while most correct, calls for a good level of professionalism by the husband and the family and should be practiced most diligently so as to avoid accidental shootings that can occur in the dark under the stress of the situation. Forewarned is forearmed. Practice reduces untimely accidents. You call the shots.

The best tactic for street survival is to force the enemy to fight on your terms, not his. Use the principle of the safe room to your advantage. Don't go hunting for your enemy if you can avoid it. You don't want to run the risk of being killed and then having the intruder go after your family. The chances of your successfully stalking and killing an armed intruder is statistically very low, some claim next to zero. Trying to be an expert in house-clearing goes against the advice of experts, who avoid this whenever possible, only attempting it with odds of up to nine against one and then being ready to accept the casualties involved in such difficult and dangerous operations.

In Israel, SWAT teams have taken to firing antitank rockets into so-called safe houses where armed killers are holed up. They have learned that even highly trained teams of specialists find room-to-room house-clearing a costly task in human lives and casualties. These experts use stun grenades, tear gas, and infrared night vision goggles—things you almost certainly don't have. However, even if you do have them, you can't be as effective as a trained team of experts.

Many times when we read about a home owner successfully doing a house-clearing job, we later find out that either his opponent was too stupid for words or our hero had a stroke of luck. These are not things to bet one's life on. Bravery alone doesn't guarantee success.

A few years back, we had some killers take over a room of a hotel in Tel Aviv. An Israeli officer passing by heard the commotion and, drawing his handgun, single-handedly decided to respond, charging into a room filled with terrorists and hostages. He was cut down in a hail of fire and died. Later, a trained SWAT team took the terrorists out. Our officer had been trained to attack, only in this case he did not have a battalion of troops and firepower behind him. Alone and in unfamiliar terrain, the brave officer simply threw his life away. Bravery alone was not enough.

The trick of surviving in the inner defense circle is to force the enemy to come to you. Make him the would-be house cleaner. Let him face those almost 100-percent odds of failure. You stay behind good cover, lie in wait; you be the ensconced armed defender and ambusher. Properly armed and having plenty of ammunition, you are in an ideal position to command a narrow approach corridor to your safe room. Now it is the intruder who must break cover, exposing himself as he negotiates narrow hallways, staircases, and open areas, all the time moving toward the deadly ambush you have prepared for him. You have the advantage—the intruder does not know where you are, if you are armed, or even if you are aware of his presence. You have the very formidable advantage of surprise. You call the shots. You didn't wander from your inner defense circle to search for the bad guy who, upon hearing your advance, would have gotten behind cover and turned the tables on you, thus becoming the ensconced defender in your castle.

Remember, the basis of the three-circle defense system is the concept of layered defense. Such a defense forces your enemy to negotiate a long and complicated series of obstacles that not only slow his advance but warn you of it.

The Interior Obstacle Course

Besides an alarm system and dogs, I like to have furniture obstacles that are so placed that someone unfamiliar with the house will bump into them, thus creating noise. Along with this, I have a step that my son liked to jump on when he came down the stairs. That step squeaks now. I've never had it fixed because I realized it is an excellent warning system, alerting me to someone moving up to the second floor where the bedrooms are.

Think of what objects you can place in someone's path that will fall, break, make noise, anything to warn you of the approach of an intruder. Such items can be placed anywhere in your outer and middle circles of defense, increasing your layered defense network, adding to it in an innovative manner.

Making It All Come Together

Novices, when facing the problem of keeping street monsters out of their homes, tend to divide security into two parts: passive security elements and a gun. They usually rely on one or the other alone. This is a gross error. Guns alone cannot provide adequate defense. Passive security alone cannot provide any. It's the marriage of the two that works. The passive security elements act as obstacles to warn you of the approach of an enemy; they slow his advance. When and if he has breached these defensives or is about to breach them, the gun can be brought into play. It is the final card, the trump card, the one you will use only after all else has failed or is about to fail and life and limb are at risk.

You Call the Police

Even if everything falls into place as you have planned, you still will call the police. Whoever calls will probably be asked by the police to stay on the line. This allows intelligence data to flow between you and the police. The responding officers are then at less risk, being less likely to be shot by you or, for that matter, shoot you. That is why it is important for the home owner not to go walking about, especially with a gun in hand.

Good tactics and common sense (think before you leap) are a winning combination. Don't separate them. Add know-how, training, and proper scenario thinking, and you should enormously increase your chances of winning against the scum that comes out of the street to invade your home.

Life Over Property

In defending your home from the entry of street predators, it is important to keep one simple fact in mind: material things can usually be replaced; you and your loved ones cannot. The first priority is the protection of human beings, not possessions.

The law does not smile upon people shooting other people for mere "property," no matter how valuable or enjoyable such property may be to you. Your weapons should be viewed as last resort protection for the saving of human life. You may disagree with such restraints, but never forget we all live in some form of organized society and are bound to the laws of that society. Following them diligently is what separates us from those that break the law out on the street.

....

STREET SURVIVAL LESSONS

1) *House weapon.* A house weapon is a must. A "hot" weapon is always superior to any "cold" weapon, but any weapon is preferable to no weapon at all.

2) *Firearms safety.* Firearms safety is an individual family matter. No two families are the same, and the subject must be closely studied so that the best plan is selected. However, some principles are universal. Never keep loaded firearms around. Store ammunition and guns separately. If you display your unloaded guns, train everyone not to touch them without your express permission.

3) *Safe rooms*. The master bedroom is the best choice unless you are a single parent. In that case, a child's room may be a better choice.

4) *Family teamwork*. Everyone should know their job.

5) *Don't be a hero*. Let the professionals go after an intruder. Your first priority is your family.

6) *Obstacle course*. Place obstacles in your home to warn you.

7) *Know police procedures*. Have a clear understanding of how to inform the police and not endanger anyone when they arrive.

Chapter Nine

Survival in Riots

*I*t is an unfortunate truth that we live in the most riot-prone times. Hardly a night goes by that we do not watch some riot or riots on TV. Riots have become an almost natural part of twentieth-century living, and I suspect the twenty-first century will be the same. With the very perceptible decrease in the standard of living around the globe has grown a distorted mirror image of civil discontent and disorder. One shudders at the thought of a real economic collapse stemming from massive, nonpayable, and steadily growing world debt that explodes into run-away inflation. The clock is ticking on life as we have known it in the past. The future is uncertain and almost certainly downhill. Riots will be part of the future, possibly mass rioting on a scale never before seen. It would be remiss to write a book on street survival and not include the phenomenon of riots. We in Israel have had more than our share of such riots. While attempting to keep politics out of our dissertation, we will study the Israeli experience. Let us delve into Israeli secrets of riot survival, bearing in mind that we are describing riots and not legitimate demonstrations, which are a right of democratic and free dissent.

USING THE PSYCHOLOGY OF RIOTERS
TO SURVIVE THE MEDIA-RIOT ALLIANCE

Riots can be based on genuine grievances or what are perceived to be grievances. Riots explode into the streets after an incident that is tied to these grievances occurs. When this happens, riot leaders will magnify the incident for their own purposes. In this work they have a willing servant: the media.

The electronic and print media usually cover this superficial aspect of the riot, sometimes using it to editorialize their own political point of view and social agenda. Riots are tailor-made for TV, giving the camera what it likes best—violent, fast-moving action in living color. Riots and the media have a very symbiotic relationship, feeding on one another. This is the riot story that most of us are subjected to in our daily diet of evening news.

But there are other aspects to riots, aspects that sometimes don't fit into the "underdog" image that the leaders of a riot and the media both want to suggest. The David (rioters) and Goliath (police) story needs the rioters to be the "good guys" and the police the "bad guys." Anything that interferes with this simplistic fairy tale is therefore usually suppressed. If something does go against the grain of the story, for instance, rioters filmed pulling someone from a truck and beating him unconscious on the street, the incident is excused as being a quasi-legitimate action of the rioters, who were driven to the action. Understanding for rioters is liberal; understanding of the problems the police face, stringent. Street survival deems that one must be conscious of this media game.

Riots also tend to be based on other things—things as eternal as human greed and hatred, the riot only being an accepted excuse (in some circles) for murder, rape, torture, and plunder. These acts, contrary to the media fairy tale, are not always carried out by frustrated innocent people driven to them. Many—but not all—riots have this evil component, this hidden agenda used by a criminal element hiding and using the other rioters as cover. We must keep in mind the fact that the very chaos of a riot lends itself to abuse by criminal or political elements ready to carry out their nefarious deeds.

The Riot Monster

People in riots tend to act as one organism, the riot becoming some moving, twisting monster that sweeps along those in it in a sea of human emotions. There is a *loss* of individuality that many find very attractive. The riot itself becomes a cloak, a cover that protects the individual

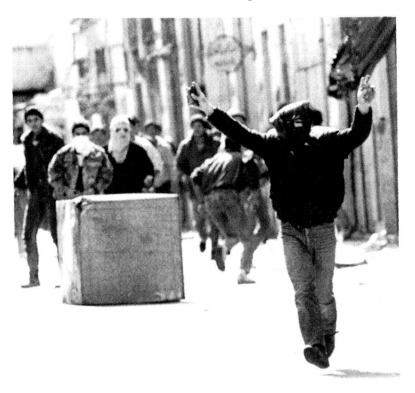

RIOT LEADER: Here we see a riot leader taunting the police as he eggs on the rioters. The riot leader is the prime target.

from being identified. Such a situation means that what the Bible calls the evil inclination comes to the surface. Rioters know that the chances of being identified, arrested, prosecuted, sentenced, and punished are slim, very slim indeed. Riots then become a convenient excuse for some humans to do everything they really wanted to do but never had the nerve to do. It's carnival time where the mask of the riot provides anonymity.

The Riot's Brain

While riots may seem totally disorganized, this is a fallacy. Riots are led by riot leaders. If you could observe a riot in a somewhat detached manner, you can find the leaders, pick them out of the crowd. They are usually at the forefront of a riot, but not always. I have seen both types of riot leaders up close as they egged on the rioters. These leaders clearly knew what they were doing. They were well versed in using the psychology of riots and rioters to their own ends. If you ever find yourself in the midst of a riot and have no means of escape, you may be able to use the psychology of a riot and rioters to survive. Schlomo Baum did just this when trapped in a riot in Gaza during a night reprisal raid carried out by Commando 101.

Case Study: Riot in Gaza

In 1953, Arab terrorists from Gaza (they were called Fedeyeen then; the PLO did not yet exist) were crossing the border each night to lay land mines in Israel. At that time Gaza was controlled by Egypt, who had captured it in Israel's 1946 War of Independence. Egyptian intelligence paid money to the Gazans for each mine laid. The death toll was rising steadily when elements of Israeli Commando 101 went over to reconnoiter the refugee camps where the bombers were being recruited.

Arik Sharon went to one camp along with four Israeli commandos, while Baum went with four others to another camp. Baum had to cross the main road and move to a large refugee camp west of it. Sharon and Baum agreed that if shooting broke out, both elements would break radio silence immediately and contact each other by walkie-talkie.

As Sharon's element penetrated the camp, they were discovered by the enemy and shot at. One of Sharon's commandos was hit. Sharon charged forward and stormed the enemy position. Meir Har-Zion, one of Israel's bravest soldiers, had his tommy gun jam up on him because they had crawled across the sand on their bellies, and the extremely fine *les* (sand) that was abundant in the area had got into the innards of his weapon.

Sharon carried an M1 carbine, and it also jammed from the microsand. He ignored it and pressed forward the attack, knowing that to do otherwise would result in their being pinned down and trapped by the superior enemy forces.

Sharon charged into an enemy position and cracked his carbine over their heads. Using such audacity and surprise, the Israelis secured the position. The wounded commando was just being pulled into the captured position when a horrible, blood-curdling roar rolled over the night sands, moving toward them like an approaching storm. Suddenly, shots rang out and bullets started to land around them like hail. A riot had broken out in the camp and was swirling toward them across the sands.

Sharon snapped on his walkie-talkie and called for help. He turned to see hundreds of rioters firing rifles and brandishing huge axes and knives as they surged out of the camp and ran toward them.

Baum didn't know the exact location of Sharon's element. He and his unit had just cut the wires of the other camp where some 6,000 Gazans lived. He did know that many of them were running to join the attack and butcher Sharon and his commandos. Screams of "Kill the Jews! Slit their throats!" filled the night. Baum had to make one of those instant decisions in battle that spell life or death. He knew that the rioters knew the exact location of Sharon's element and he didn't. So he joined them! Shouting to his men to stay close and "follow me" (the command of Israeli officers in battle), Baum led his commandos into the mob as he yelled in perfect Arabic: "Kill the Jews! Slit their throats!"

The swirling mass of angry rioters moved down the dark, narrow lanes of the camp, lit only by a thin sliver of moonlight. As they moved forward, the enormous crowd of rioters was compacted into ever-narrowing dark alleyways. The buildings almost seemed to be closing in on them. Baum and his four commandos were being pressed inside of an armed mob of 300 rioters. Trapped!

Baum now knew the direction they were moving and where Sharon and his men were located. He looked around as the rioters swirled ahead and saw that his men were with him, still undetected by the frenzied rioters who were being spurred on by their leaders. Baum made a decision to confuse the rioters and use the opportunity to break through to Sharon. He ordered, "Open fire!" All the tommy guns opened up at once, the heavy .45 bullets making a loud smack as they slammed into rioters and riot leaders, cutting a corridor through them as they charged, Baum at point, one commando on the right, another on the left, then one each right and left again. The Israeli commandos fired 15 to 20 rounds each in short bursts. This had a devastating effect on the armed rioters who were mowed down by a hail of heavy bullets from the Thompsons. Accurate firepower had opened an avenue for Baum and his men. They rushed through it. Thirty rioters lay dead and another 40 wounded.

"Follow me!" shouted Baum as he charged in the direction of where Sharon and his men lay trapped. As the Israelis moved down the dark alley, it continued into a new construction site, getting narrower and narrower until it was only 2 yards across, lined with Mideastern windows that rose a half-meter from street level to a height of almost 2 meters. Suddenly, they heard the tell-tale sound of a Bren gun opening up, spitting out a deadly stream of bullets across the alley. Trapped again!

Baum motioned for his men to stop. He went to the ground and slowly crawled along the wall until he was right below the window from where the Bren was firing. He wanted to throw a grenade, but being "street wise," he knew that what seemed so evident might not be as easy as it appeared.

He reached up and felt something. An antigrenade net had been stretched across the window. He smiled to himself, knowing that if he had tossed that grenade up into the window it would have bounced back into his lap and exploded, probably killing him and some of his men. Baum reached up into his backpack for one of his two "Eliov bottles."

(Eliov was a Jewish scientist who fought against the Nazis from deep in Russia to Berlin. When there, he deserted the Red Army and joined the soldiers of the Jewish Brigade, a Palestinian-Jewish unit in the British army. What Eliov did was vastly improve the Molotov cocktail. He invented a new formula and design that used a deadly blend of diesel fuel, gasoline, aluminum dust, and sliced rubber crepe from the soles of shoes that would melt from the intense heat and stick to any target hit. A top-secret ingredient was also added, one that is still held secret to this very day. This was all put into a very thin-walled glass bottle that was developed and made in Israel for this specific task. It sported a long, thin neck for easy grasping and a grenade-type pin that activated the contents seconds after being pulled.)

Pulling the pin, Baum slammed the Eliov bottle up and into the screen. The dark alley was illuminated in an intense white light as the Eliov bottle exploded, roaring into intense flames that caused a type of vacuum that sucked the flames into the dark room where the Bren gunners were still firing.

The machine gun fire stopped abruptly, and the screaming gunners rolled around in agony or ran berserk from the blazing inferno.

Baum jumped forward and opened up with his Thompson. Within seconds, it was all over. The five-man Bren crew lay dead. The way to the rescue of Sharon and his team was open. Baum led his men forward, shouting for Sharon. His shouts were answered, and the two units joined forces. They turned to see that the rioters had reorganized and were moving forward fast in another mass attack. The wounded commando lay in pain, his femur shattered. Four men would be needed to carry him through the desert and back into Israeli territory. Baum knew he had to buy them some time. He made an instant decision to counterattack the swirling mob that was bearing down on them. He had to gain 5 to 7 minutes for the others. This he did, personally killing another 30 to 40 armed rioters as he dodged a deadly shower of enemy bullets. The commando force reached the Israeli lines in safety. Not a man was lost.

Interview with Lt. Col. Schlomo Baum

E.S.: Do you think any combat lesson learned in this raid would pertain to survival in the streets?

S.B.: Absolutely. You are perfectly correct in your premise that the principles of combat are the same whether we are speaking of warfare or street survival. It's time we relearned that fact.

E.S.: What street survival lessons did you learn from the raid?

S.B.: A riot is a riot. It is usually a very confused situation, especially if it occurs at night. My idea to join the riot in its early stage, blending into it, was probably the most critical decision I made. It helped us escape and find our buddies. We used the riot and were not made victims by it. If you are ever trapped by a riot in some urban center, this idea just might save your life. If it is possible and all escape routes are closed to you, it may he better to take the audacious decision and actually risk joining the rioters rather than to stand out like a sore thumb and have them turn against you.

E.S.: How did you make that decision so quickly?

S.B.: Experience has taught me to make instant decisions. This is one of the keys to being a good commander of men and also to survive in combat. As I said before, never concentrate only on one thing. You also have to think simultaneously about the next step you plan to take. Be one step ahead of your opponent.

E.S.: Would scenario planning help give those of us without your vast combat experience some of these skills?

S.B.: Yes. I use the technique of preplanning as much as possible.

STREET SURVIVAL LESSONS

1) *Riot leaders.* Most riots are organized and are not the leaderless mob that is usually portrayed in the media. Even if they do start out in a spontaneous manner, leadership comes to the forefront in short order.

2) *Trapped in a moving riot.* The tactics of an individual trapped in a moving riot should be either to outrun the rioters or, if undiscovered, to join them in a clandestine manner, at least until an escape can be attempted.

3) *Don't be captured.* To fall into the hands of a mob of rioters could be a death sentence. Rioters are in a highly emotional state. Being spotted and captured is therefore to be avoided at all costs.

Case Study: My Personal Riot Story Outside of Schem, Israel
Years ago, I had a teaching commitment that turned out to be a learning experience for me. One day, I was supposed to drive up to the north of Israel to visit the Israeli Army NCO school when riots broke out all over Judea, Samaria, and Gaza. The army warned us that the safest way to get north was by the coastal route and not by going up the center of the country through Arab towns and villages.

I told my driver there was no way we were taking the long way, and we turned directly north and moved up the center of the country. About two hours from my house, we came upon black smoke rising into the sky about a half-mile ahead of us. The road we were on was not the modern super coastal highway but rather a narrow asphalt one in the mountains. I knew the smoke was probably from tires being burned in the village up ahead. Within a minute or two, we turned a bend in the road and came upon Israeli cars that were blocked by heavy boulders that had been rolled onto the road, as well as some burning tires. The Israelis in the trapped cars immediately started shouting, "An officer! An officer!" I ordered the driver to pull over and got out to see about 40 rioters who were on the roof of an unfinished building some 60 yards from the road. They were hurling rocks the size of baseballs upon the hapless cars and their owners. A young man in a red shirt seemed to be the riot leader. When he spotted me, he got even more excited, waving his arms and shouting for more rocks. Within seconds, the shower of rocks turned into a hail storm.

I ordered my driver to stay with the cars and cover me with his M16 but not to fire unless I ordered him to. I then told the trapped car owners and their passengers to get off their duffs and clear the road. This they proceeded to do immediately. At that time, a few years before what is now called the Intifada broke out, my orders were correct. This is not true today, when rioters have taken to booby-trapping road barricades.

Pulling my Swenson 1911 from my military holster, I made for the building where the rioters were. Large rocks and iron bars whizzed past my head, and I realized I'd better do something quick or I'd get my brains splattered. I stopped about 40 yards from the rioters and took careful aim at the roof's edge where the leader in the red shirt was standing. Aiming about 2 inches under his big toe, I fired one shot and blew a large chunk out of the edge of the roof. I knew that Swenson was more accurate than I could shoot and wouldn't let me down if I did my part. Everything suddenly got very quiet. The rocks stopped. The mob moved back from the edge of the roof. I later found out the reason for this. It seems at that time most Israeli soldiers only fired warning shots in the air, and this was a new experience for the rioters. I turned back toward the car and immediately saw my driver jumping up and down shouting for me to turn around. I did so and saw the mob surging forward, pouring from the building as rocks filled the sky, some only missing me by inches.

The riot leader had taken off his red shirt and was waving

it over his head like some flag, spurring the rioters on. He was on the edge of that roof again, his foot sticking out halfway into space. I took careful aim, squeezed the trigger, and cracked the cinder block directly under his foot. At this he panicked, convinced that I was one hell of a bad shot who was getting luckier and luckier by the second. The rioters retreated and the roof was cleared. I made it back to my driver, backpedaling slowly, the .45 covering my movement. By this time, the burning tires had been pulled off the road and the boulders were clear. The driver was standing alone; the cars had left. As we got into our car, I turned to see the bare-chested riot leader run to the edge of the roof, screaming abuse at me. I unfortunately gave in to a primitive urge (which Baum later criticized me for) and gave him "the finger." This drove the riot leader so wild I could only calm him down by once again taking careful aim with the Swenson. This definitely seemed to cool his ardor, and he jumped back from the roof's edge.

We got into our car and leisurely drove toward the NCO school on a trip that was thereafter uneventful, except that I noticed a car driven by an Israeli security man and flagged him down, informing him of what had transpired. He got on his radio and phoned in a report of the incident.

We arrived at the school late, and I apologized to the base commander, a big, blond paratroop colonel who told me he knew the spot well, having laid an ambush there only a week or two before. He had sent in a decoy team of a few men, which confronted the rioters while a second group of paratroopers ambushed them from behind, doing good work with their billy clubs so as to turn them away from their potentially deadly habits.

When I arrived back at headquarters, I filed a report of the incident with my commander, Col. G., who wanted to know why I hadn't followed standing orders on opening fire into the air when faced with rioters. I told him my Hebrew wasn't too good and I missed that part. He stared at me for a moment, frowned, then slowly grinned, nodding for me to get the hell out of his office.

STREET SURVIVAL LESSONS

1) *Target the riot leader.* Always try to engage the riot leader rather than individual rioters. It is the best way to turn a riot in another direction or break it up. If you are forced to fire and aim to hit, it saves lives since you "cut off the head of the snake."

2) *Don't turn your back on a riot.* Never do a stupid thing like turning your back on any potential danger, thinking it has ceased. Move back fast and cover your retreat. Making yourself a tempting target serves to embolden your adversary.

3) *Call your shots.* Never shoot to kill if your life is not in danger. I did not feel my life was in danger at the time. Since then, I have had time to see the effects of such riots. I am not so sure I would have shot below his big toe a second time.

4) *Act professional.* If you are a police officer or soldier called in to face a rioting mob, do your job with professional dignity. Don't demean yourself and your uniform by stooping to the level of the mob. (Do not make obscene gestures.)

5) *Know your skill level.* Taking what some would call a long distance shot with a difficult goal in mind, namely, hitting just under the riot leader's foot, was not a foolhardy or reckless thing to do. I knew the level of my skill. I knew the proven accuracy of my weapon.

6) Backup. Do have someone cover your back with a firearm if you go forward against the riot. Backup is important. If you have it, use it.

WHO SAYS WORDS CAN'T KILL?

I know of many deaths here in Israel that can be traced to the individual's refusing to defend himself because he thinks such an act can get him into trouble with the law. This is especially true when the press is unfriendly to weapons use by the potential victim in his legitimate self-defense. An unfriendly press helps cast fear into gun users by falsely and deliberately labeling such people aggressors. One case of such unfriendly and grossly biased press coverage comes to mind.

Case Study: Right-Wing Murderer at Jaffa Gate

The old city quarter of Jerusalem is visited by hundreds of thousands of tourists a year, being the area where sites holy to Judaism, Christianity, and Islam stand side by side. It was then perfectly normal for an Israeli couple in their 60s to be at one of the gates of the old city, the Jaffa gate, as they drove back from visiting the Western Wall of the Second Temple.

It was early in the morning, and the woman was hungry, so she stopped to buy a roll from one of the bread cart vendors who sell such things to passersby. Suddenly, a horrible piercing scream shattered the pastoral scene. The husband turned to see his wife running from the bread cart, the Arab vendor in hot pursuit, waving a large bread knife over his head. She jumped into the waiting car. The knife-wielder slashed at the husband, who pulled a Beretta .22 LR-caliber pistol and shot him a few times. The knife wielder fell to the ground, mortally wounded.

A headline in the press that night proclaimed, "Arab Murdered by Israeli in Old City." The article told of the Israeli's past history, alluding to the fact that he was a member of the right-wing Jewish underground (the Irgun) during Israel's fight for independence decades before. It also said that the knife-wielder had a known history of mental illness, having been hospitalized on two occasions, alluding to the idea that he therefore was not responsible for the attack, which could have been handled in some other, less violent manner.

No newspaper ever questioned the fact that a known mental case with a history of violence was allowed back onto the streets. The perpetrator was turned into the victim. The victims of the attack were turned into the perpetrators, a situation much like we see in many newspapers across the globe.

STREET SURVIVAL LESSON

1) *You will be bad-mouthed.* Be prepared for negative press if you use a firearm in self-defense. The press seems bent on portraying any act of self-defense with a firearm as akin to murderous aggression. Still, better a negative headline than a head cut off by a bread knife.

FOREWARNED IS FOREARMED

Riots do not occur in vacuums. Those trained to watch for such things can see the signs of pressure buildup. The warning signs can help you avoid riot-prone areas or at least put you on the alert so that you and your family can be in a position to survive. The following are some things to look out for and precautions to take.

Tell-Tale Signs

Look for a series of incidents portrayed by the popular press as deliberate mistreatment of a minority or segment of the population, even when such portrayal is unjustified. The press is actually building up a head of steam (whether deliberately or not is irrelevant) that will certainly explode into a full-blown riot. When this explosion will occur is difficult to predict, but being aware of what is happening around you at least puts you on guard. Look upon these incidents as you would earth tremors. The tremors warn you of an impending earthquake. Which one of these tremors will turn into the big quake is hard to know, but you have been forewarned.

Be especially leery of hot weather. Hot weather likes riots, especially when the media justify the hot weather as an excuse for one. I remember a liberal friend of mine trying to justify a riot that occurred in a neighborhood of walk-up tenement apartments as being justified and not the fault of the rioters. "Imagine living up there in the heat and humidity," he lamented. "Can you blame any human being for rioting under those conditions?" When I reminded him that we both had grown up and lived in these flats many years back and that the weather was just as hot and humid then, he looked quite dumbstruck. The thought had never crossed his mind. I went on to inform him we never ran into the street attacking cars or smashing storefronts. He just stared. He seemed at a loss for words by the logic of what I said.

Unfortunately, logic never seems to win over emotion when people make false excuses for criminal acts. This is intellectually dishonest if nothing else.

No News is Bad News

Another factor that can be used to trigger a riot is the need for a big story on TV. Expanding a small incident into a big story is a basic tactic of the media when the news is devoid of any real interest. That such a ploy triggers a riot is not seen as a misdeed of the media but only as a manifestation of a healthy and free press. Journalistic responsibility is sometimes cast aside in the quest for higher ratings or sales.

Car Radio On

I would suggest always keeping the car radio tuned to a local station when driving. Sometimes the first warnings of riots are broadcast on radio, especially local talk shows. Not entering a potential riot zone is the very best way of surviving a riot.

Observe the Abnormal

Be aware of activity that is happening in the street around you, and don't ignore what seems to be abnormal activity, such as cars stopped and people milling about, especially when the people look law-abiding and are trying to signal something to you.

A few years back, one of my neighbors was driving along the coastal highway here in Israel, an area deemed very safe by those who believe in such things in this day and age. They came to many cars that were bunched up and saw people trying to flag them down. The father, believing that a car accident had occurred up ahead and not wanting to be held up by traffic, slipped by the cars and drove into a group of terrorists who were spraying the area with submachine gun fire. They had landed on the coast. The father swerved around, but it was too late. Bullets slammed into the car and hit his son, who was in the back seat. They got away, but their son was hit in the throat. His mother tried to stop the bleeding. He slowly died in her arms.

Copters and Sirens
Be aware of helicopters flying low overhead, especially when you hear police sirens in the area. This may be a sign that something is amiss. That something could be an accident or a VIP driving through, but then again, it could be a riot or a street shoot-out. Like the alley cat, never turn off your sensitivity to your environment, even if you are in your air-conditioned sports car. Life still goes on around you, and sometimes that life is dangerous to your health and well-being.

Big Brother
To survive street riots, one must not only be well armed and have street savvy but understand the attitudes of one's own government as well. Even if people have firearms, the fear of governmental punishment may force some not to use them, even as legitimate self-defense. Fear of Big Brother government is not theoretical anymore. It is a living reality. It is as important a factor in street survival as that punk you meet in the parking lot. Why do governments have such negative attitudes about legitimate self-defense? Let's try to unravel this mystery.

Governmental Deceit
A phenomenon of our times seems to be an increasing

trend of governments lying to their own people. Budget figures are doctored. National debt payments are deemed assets rather than liabilities. Assassinations of national figures by shadowy groups are labeled the deed of a lone, deranged murderer who is then conveniently done away with so that no public trial takes place. The thieving murderous behavior of rioters is excused in the name of liberalism when the real reason is political expediency by elected officials who are afraid of losing power. Everything and everyone but the rioter is blamed. Even the inanimate object becomes suspect. Even guns are deemed guilty of committing crimes rather than criminals. Reality is cast aside as elected officials and their lackeys spin webs of deceit so as to cling to political power. The politician's job, rather than the victim, is what is all-important, and if standing up for the truth jeopardizes that job, the truth (and the public) be damned.

Here in Israel, elements of the press and some politicians deemed the tossing of stones at passing cars not life-threatening. Working as a newspaper columnist, I openly criticized this attitude. Stones are not marshmallows, I wrote. The number of Israelis with permanent brain damage who were struck by stones can attest to that. Stones are not pebbles but rather large rocks that kill. The stone has killed more than its share of people since the dawn of history, whether it was shot from a sling, tied to a stick, or tossed by hand.

Case Study: He Who Hesitates is Lost

Two cases come to mind that illustrate the point of political and press-manipulated fear of illegal use of firearms. The second of these cases resulted in an unnecessary death.

A few months ago, an Israeli settler fired his handgun at an Arab who attacked him. The Arab subsequently died. It seems the Arab had illegally trespassed and was allowing his large herd of sheep and goats to feed on lands owned and cultivated by the settlement. When ordered to move off with his herd, the Arab attacked the settler and was shot. Upon the arrival of the police, the Israeli's handgun was confiscated and a hullabaloo hit the press about how the Israeli was in deep trouble with the law for firing his legal weapon in self-defense. Political leftists and some elements of the press called him a murderer.

I remember that it was only a matter of a week before another such incident occurred, not very far from the previous incident. Only this time when the Arab moved his animals onto private land and challenged the settler, the Israeli hesitated and did not draw his weapon. He was knifed by his attacker. He didn't get into trouble with the law. He just lost his life.

One does not have to ban firearms to restrict their legitimate use. Self-serving bureaucrats and politicians allied with elements of the media can make it extremely difficult for law-abiding citizens. This, of course, is not to claim that every politician, bureaucrat, or newsman thinks this way, but the effects of even a small, vocal minority can cost innocent lives.

....

STREET SURVIVAL LESSON

1) *He who hesitates is lost.* Do not hesitate to use your weapon when you and your loved ones face mortal danger. Don't cower in the face of those who try to reverse reality in the quest to achieve their own self-serving agenda.

....

HOW TO BREAK THE WEAKEST POINT OF A RIOT

Try to find the leader or leaders of the riot and, if forced to open fire, target them, wounding or killing them if need be. As I said before, the old adage about cutting off the head of the snake applies in spades when you fall victim to a riot.

Riots can be composed of hundreds and even thousands of rioters, and unless you have a truck full of ammo at your beck and call, you will have to call your shots. Aim at the leaders of the riot and score hits. Even if you can't find the real higher-ups, you will find that in every front line or behind it there is usually a subleader who seems to be controlling the shouting or the throwing of Molotov cocktails, etc. These persons qualify as leaders and should be prime targets. Eliminate them either by deliberate wounding or fatal fire, and the area of the riot you are personally concerned with resembles a headless snake that writhes about out of control—making it less of a danger. You will have broken its strongest point and made it leaderless.

To accomplish this task, you will have to be cool and expert in your marksmanship and be capable of hitting a target up to and even beyond 100 yards. While being a firm advocate of point fire, like all professionals I am also a true believer in the art of aimed fire when time, distance, and circumstances allow. This includes long-distance handgun shooting (with your street-carry handgun, not one of those "pocket rifles" so popular with long-distance handgun sport shooters today).

Long-distance handgun shooting with your carry gun is a needed skill in riot survival, one that must be practiced in a very diligent manner so that it becomes a normal part of your self-defense repertoire. It's nice to have a good rifle as your primary weapon, but this should never be your sole means of engaging long-distance targets. Always have at least one handgun along that can do this job, just in case something happens to your long gun.

Case Study: Night Training at Base "X"

I remember having a platoon of paratroopers at a training base somewhere in Samaria, Israel. They were armed with M16 rifles, which in those days had the flip-up peep sights on them, the first for 0 to 300 meters and the second for the longer distance of 350 meters. Some "expert" had been trying to eliminate the long-distance sight, saying it was not needed for combat and most shooters couldn't hit with it anyway. They wanted to turn it into a night sight, drilling a big hole in it and ruining it in the process. This I adamantly disagreed with. Unfortunately, the paratroopers had got wind of the negative idea that you could not hit targets at long range with the M16 (then new in the army) and were standing about in a most nonsupportive manner when I

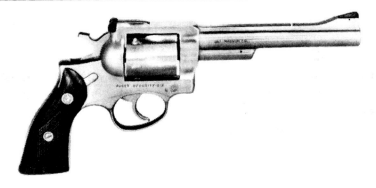

RUGER SECURITY SIX: I used a blue model with a 9mmP factory-fitted cylinder for my "circus act."

pointed to a barrel target at some 370 meters, which they were supposed to engage with the long sight. That it was night and the only light was a small can containing a kerosene-soaked rag (Israelis call them *goozneekim*) flickering at the 370 range didn't help matters. I realized that it was time for what I jokingly told my wife Cynthia was my "circus act."

I used to carry along a special Ruger Security Six with a 6-inch barrel that a friend at Ruger had fitted with an interchangeable 9mmP cylinder. It shot very accurately and accepted Uzi submachine gun ammo with no problems. Half-moon clips helped in fast loading and unloading.

I walked over to a sandbag wall that I had constructed. It provided the shooter with support and cover and was used in engaging the long-distance targets. When I pulled out the Ruger, I could hear mumbling in the background as the platoon viewed my antics. Opening the cylinder, I dispensed with the half-moon clips filled with ball ammo and instead placed a single tracer round in one of its chambers, knowing that I had to hit that barrel with the first shot. It had to be spectacular; anything else wouldn't have had the desired psychological effect. Bracing my elbows on the parapet of that

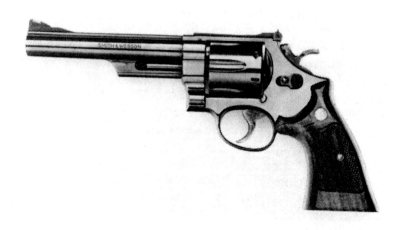

S&W MODEL 29: An excellent third handgun that fills the roll of a long gun when one is not available.

military position, I cocked back the hammer, then reckoned how much front sight I needed to hold onto that barrel, which I could hardly see, even with the light of the burning kerosene. I had been shooting lots of targets with that Ruger and knew the gun well, but still that tracer was not what you'd call target accurate and had missed on the first shot many a time, even with better ammo.

I proceeded to say a little prayer as I slowly squeezed the trigger. We were greeted with a loud bang and a fiery flash as the tracer exited the gun barrel and began what seemed an almost leisurely arc across the darkness to the target, poorly illuminated by the flickering kerosene-soaked rags. The tracer bullet plunged into the center of the barrel and a shower of sparks exploded, lighting up the darkness. I turned to those young paratroopers, who cheered and patted me on the back. The gamble had paid off. Maybe some angel was standing there beside me. Anyway, they said if I could do that with a pistol, they would be ashamed if they couldn't do it with a rifle. From then on, the long sight on the M16 was left alone to do what it was designed for—hit targets at 350 meters and beyond.

Long-Distance Handgunning at Rioters

The first thing in understanding the art of long-distance pistol shooting is accepting the fact that it is a normal part of everyday work with a handgun and not some special skill that only select handgunners can learn. Over the years, one thing that amazed me was the adamant rejection of the idea's feasibility by those who had never even tried it. I have used this skill not only in a riot situation but in the psychological context of eliminating opposition to some of my somewhat radical (at the time) ideas of mass training an army. I found there was nothing like hitting a small target at hundreds of yards with a carry handgun to make friends and influence people. I carried the long-distance shooting skills of the men of the Wild West as taught by Elmer Keith to the Wild East, where they are now rooted and growing.

Though we are now speaking of learning the use of this skill on riot leaders, we, of course, can think of other scenarios for its use in street survival. Examples include a crazed person firing from a rooftop, an urban terrorist who has opened up on hapless passersby, drive-by killers who have fired at you and are now racing away, and so on. The scenarios are almost endless.

Short-Barreled Cannon

The first rule is to view our handgun as a short-barreled howitzer. It is much harder for a howitzer to place a shell shot in a rain barrel at 3 miles than for you to hit a man at 150 yards, yet we accept the capability of the howitzer doing this much more readily than the handgun. The rules of artillery fire are basic to the use of this "small artillery piece" called the handgun.

Stable Position

First, you must get into a stable position. Obviously, if you are unstable you will not be able to hit seemingly pinpoint targets at what are considered absurdly long ranges for a handgun. The most stable positions are the Creedmore prone position and the braced sitting position. Unfortunately, you should not assume these sporting positions when you are in a riot or combat situation. They are excellent when your target is a rock or a deer. Using such a position when facing armed adversaries is a formula for disaster and cuts your chances for street survival by many percentile points. You must therefore use positions that give you as much support and cover as possible while still retaining your ability to respond to attacks that may come at you from the flanks or behind. When Keith popularized the fine art of long-distance pistol shooting, he did not have combat in mind but hunting. The positions the combat shooter must take are quite different.

Standing, Standing Braced Positions

Standing out there in the street is not a good idea. Sure, I took a chance when facing the rioters on the flat roof of that building, but I was looking for a psychological effect on the rioters and was not interested in killing. Did I commit an error? Possibly. I could have been killed by a rock, or one of them could have shot me. I was more lucky than smart. I learned from that bit of foolishness and won't repeat my mistake.

Whenever possible, try to get behind cover and move into a braced position for more stability and, hence, more accurate fire. You may have to forget about how to place your feet. You probably won't find the ideal level ground of a shooting range anyway. Try not to get into a strained position if you can help it, though you may find that you simply have no choice. Usually, your feet will get into the best position they can; after all, that's what they've been doing for you all your life. The same with breathing or the lack of it. Don't overemphasize breathing control; it will come to you naturally as you aim. Concentrate on the target, sight picture, and trigger control—and on not getting ambushed as you do it.

I find the Weaver (of course, Fitzgerald at Colt did it before) hold works best for this task in any of its slight variations. Some may prefer isosceles. Use any support, turning it into the braced standing position by leaning into it with your shoulder. (Be careful not to touch the handgun against any support you use with this or any position.)

You can also shoot over the support by resting your arms on it, but this makes you a target. Don't do it unless no other choice exists.

Kneeling, Kneeling Braced Positions

I find the kneeling or kneeling braced position enables you to quickly engage targets that may come out of nowhere while you are concentrating on one at long range. Because of this, this position (and its variations) is a good one when facing targets of the two-legged variety.

Rollover Prone Position

The classic rollover prone position that was perfected in IPSC shooting works out in the street, especially if you don't have good cover and have been pinned down by enemy fire or don't want to rise, thus exposing yourself to detection.

ONE BULLET, ONE ENEMY

We are speaking of the use of the handgun against enemy targets at long range. Enemies who are bent on killing you are probably better armed than you are. Because of this, zeroing in shots against your adversaries may not be possible because they will warn them of your intentions and position, enabling them to take appropriate counteraction. Another problem is the fact that in battle you may not be able to see the bullet's impact, hitting in a near-miss pattern, which you would normally use for bullet correction when shooting for sport. You may only have that one shot, so learn to make it count. Practice making only one long-distance shot at any target and not two, three, or more. Anything less is just not practical in combat. Can it be done? Yes. Can it be done most of the time? Yes, if you really get a feel for your handgun and its cartridge.

Know Your Cartridge

To be proficient in the art of long-distance street shooting with the handgun, one must spend time learning the trajectory of the load selected for the task. This, coupled with the knowledge of how much front sight to hold above the bottom of the rear sight notch so as to hit our target at different ranges, forms the basis of street survival with the handgun. However, all of this will count for naught if you do not do other things in a correct and professional manner. That is why it is very important to use bullets that are of the same weight and cartridges that fire them at roughly the same velocity. Mixing up different weight bullets and different powered cartridges is a very good way to mess up your chances for hitting pinpoint targets at long range. Violating the principle of uniformity may move the bullet's point of impact, and you will sadly pay by most probably missing your long-range target.

Getting a Grip on Things

Obtaining a good solid grip on your handgun is very important for accurate, controlled fire at any range. I believe that handguns, be they revolvers or semiautomatics, should be gripped as high in the hand as possible. This greatly reduces felt recoil and allows for faster, controlled follow-up shots.

Hold the handgun firmly. A loose grip leads to very poor handgun control. In combat, the convulsive grip is the norm and will be the way you grip the handgun, probably without even realizing it. This is excellent with point shooting but must be moderated if at all possible for pinpoint fire at long-range targets. Still, it beats a sloppy, weak grip anytime. And again, it is the grip you will probably be using, like it or not.

For long-distance fire, the weak hand serves to brace and stabilize the shooting hand, grasping it in a firm hold, fingers over fingers, weak hand forefinger pressed underneath and up against the trigger guard.

Trigger Control

Here is where most shooters fall down; squeezing the trigger with a smooth and consistent motion takes practice—lots of it. Do it until it becomes second nature, and the skill will never leave you. I used to tell the soldiers to squeeze the trigger like a lemon, wanting to avoid a squirt in the eye, which comes from jerking or squeezing it with too much force. I'd make believe it was a lemon, and they'd almost see that squirt of lemon juice going up into my eye as I squinted. Then I'd do it more slowly, without the squint. Such theatrics may look silly, but students remember them. To this day, I'm stopped on the street by soldiers and civilians who smile and remind me to "squeeze the trigger like a lemon." They also remind me, "one bullet, one enemy."

Combat Sight Picture

Zeroing in for long-range fire is impractical since you aren't a hunter of animals but rather one of men. If you have an adjustable rear sight, it must be zeroed in for the ranges from which men may most likely attack you. I use a 25-yard battle sight zero. This puts the sights on target from 0 to about 80 yards, more or less. It makes no sense to have your sights adjusted for, say, 300 yards. While we want to be capable of long-distance handgunning, never compromise your handgun's practical accuracy at more mundane and realistic ranges to achieve it. Leaf rear sights, ultra-high front sights with range graduations, and handgun telescopes all have their place in the sporting field, not in the killing fields. Keep your sighting system strong and simple. Learn to use combat sights for long-distance targets and you will then be able to handle all targets at all practical ranges. A compromise? Of course, but a realistic one.

STREET SURVIVAL LESSONS

1) *Accurate long-range fire with a handgun.* Know the uses of long-distance pistol shooting. Do not look upon a riot as a homogeneous mass, but rather as an organism that has a head. The head is the riot leader. Try to find and eliminate him if your life is threatened. To accomplish this task, you may have to fire a long-distance handgun shot.

2)   *Keep sport and combat apart.* Never use sporting or hunting positions in combat; they are a sure-fire way to get you killed. This goes for riots, too.

3)   *One bullet, one enemy.* Learn to make that first shot count. In combat or riots, you may not have time for a second or third shot. More than one shot may compromise your concealment.

4)   *Riot handgun.* In a riot, a handgun, if handled by someone who has mastered the art of long-distance pistol shooting, can act like a long gun. Know how to do this, since chances are that if trapped in a riot, your handgun may be the only gun available.

....

Case Study: You Don't Have to Be a Victim
Bruce (my friend from Tekoa who made the bedspring barrier) just called and thanked me for his being alive. He said that my advice (which he at first had rejected) had just saved his life.

It seems an Israeli army doctor, Baruch Goldstein, had just shot up the mosque in Abraham's Tomb (over the Cave of Machpela in Hebron). Bruce had been on the road when the report came in over his radio (he kept his radio on as he had been advised to), and within minutes, rioting had broken out.

E.S.: Where were you at the time?

B: I was near the junction where the isolated side road led to my settlement of Tekoa. There was an army roadblock, and I asked if the road was open and safe. They told me it was.

E.S.: Did you believe them?

B: No. You told me never to believe anyone.

E.S.: Good. How could they know that for sure? Never bet your life on such statements. What did you do next?

B: I swung onto the road to Tekoa and drove at moderate speed with my windows open, being alert at all times to everything.

E.S.: Very good. How were you armed? Were you still insisting on carrying that Ruger Black Hawk .357 Magnum with five bullets in it?

B: Yes, but I added an M16 with five 30-round banana clips, all loaded and on me.

E.S.: I'm proud of you. What happened next? Were they waiting a few miles up the road like I predicted weeks before?

B: Yes. As I approached an Arab village, I noticed a car with four men in it. They were dressed like Hamas. They stared at me.

E.S.: What did you do then?

B: I stared back, slowed down, and poked the muzzle of the M16 out the window, just like you said I should. I looked like one mean-ass settler. They gunned the engine and roared away.

E.S.: Was there an ambush up ahead? Around the bend when you entered the village?

B: There sure as hell was. If I had gone fast I would have slammed into a road barrier made up of a metal light pole, rocks, burning tires, and barrels. Instead, I could control the car as I came under a shower of rocks from about 30 rioters.

E.S.: Did those Hamas guys get behind you like I said they might?

B: No. I think when they saw me they decided to pass on this one and drove back to Hebron. I debussed and started to make a hole in the barricade. It might have been booby-trapped, but I was worried about my wife at home. It took me 10 minutes to make an opening, all the time shooting at them to break up their rock-throwing charges. I looked and acted like Rambo, just like you told me, even though I was scared shitless. It worked. I'm home and alive. I think I got a few of them. Oh, I fired three shots signaling for help. Like you said, it was heard but no one came. Seems there was a lot of shooting going on at the time. I was on my own. Like I said, many thanks. I'm alive.

NOTE: One of Bruce's fellow settlers had been murdered

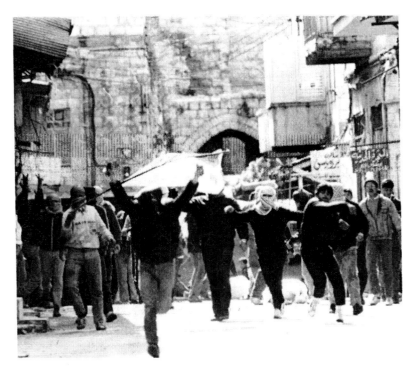

A TYPICAL INTIFADA ROADBLOCK: Woe be to anyone falling into the hands of this mob.

in a drive-by shooting only a few weeks before. His mutilated body was found in his car. He was reaching for the glove compartment, where he kept his high-capacity pistol.

After that incident, Bruce called and asked me how to drive on that isolated road. He followed the advice. He survived.

Case Study: Secret Background to the Intifada

Probably the longest-playing riot in recent memory is what the world calls the Intifada. Supposedly, this riot was triggered by an Israeli driver who accidentally ran an Arab down in Gaza. Rumors spread through Gaza that the driver had done this deliberately. Now for a rumor to be believed, the receivers of the rumor must accept the plausibility of it.

Since just such acts were being perpetrated on Israelis by Arabs, the rumor was believed.

A background story that has never appeared in print before and is probably only known by a few dozen people is that the coming of the Intifada was predicted accurately some five years before the accident in Gaza that triggered it in 1987.

It was 1982, and I was at home when the phone rang and Baum asked if I could come to his house immediately. Since he did not tell me why on the phone, I suspected it was something serious that he wanted to keep under his hat. When I got there, I was ushered into his living room, where I met a middle-aged man who I was informed was an expert on terrorism. After some pleasantries were exchanged, Baum stunned me by informing me that, in his opinion, in about five years a great general uprising of the Arabs in Judea, Samaria (so-called West Bank), and the Gaza district would break out with dire political consequences for Israel. Baum believed that the bad world press generated by the uprising (the Intifada) would damage and weaken Israel politically and result in the false conclusion that the "territories" liberated by Israel after it was attacked by Egypt, Syria, and Jordan in the Six Day War, were an obstacle to peace and would have to be abandoned. Baum assured us that such an act would put our very survival as a nation in doubt. We would find ourselves in a very dangerous position in any future war.

Because of this, Baum wanted a special unit to be established which would be made up of full-time professionals who would be highly skilled in riot control. Such a unit would spring into action when the Intifada broke out. Its mission: to squelch it within 72 hours. Baum stressed that if the riot leaders saw the riot go on beyond this short time frame, it would be a sign to them that the mass rioting could be sustained for years, slowly cracking Israel's psychological defenses, possibly leading to a Palestinian state led by Yasser Arafat, the head of the PLO.

Baum turned to me and asked if I would agree to train

such a group of experts. It would especially be important that each and every one of them be crack shots. I said that I would. Baum cautioned me to hear him out, for what he was asking for had very serious problems as far as training and mission were concerned. The select group would begin with two companies of picked marksman. They would not be allowed to shoot to kill any rioter except in the most extreme circumstances. Simply cutting down rows of rioters could be done easily by machine guns and did not call for highly skilled specialists. This, however, could not be done by Western-oriented and democratic Israel.

What was needed were snipers who would work in mass, hitting the armed rioters with crippling but not killing shots. Baum estimated that about 1,800 rioters would have to be shot in those first 72 hours. This, he believed, would stop the tactics of mass rioting in its tracks, squelch the Intifada, and save us all from much more numerous and deadly casualty figures for both Israelis and Arabs in future years.

Baum asked if I would be willing to go into the midst of riots that were now taking place in Ramallah and which he believed were only the beginning of a series of dress rehearsals of things to come. I would be assisted by a paratroop Lt. Colonel nicknamed "Mootzee" and three or four of his young security experts. My mission would be to study the feasibility of producing experts in riot control with the aforementioned mission as our goal. The unit would be in the uniforms of the Israeli Border Patrol, nominally under the Ministry of Police, but would actually take orders from the Ministry of Defense. Baum wanted to know if I thought such a project was technically possible and if I would still be interested in joining such a venture? I, of course, assured him I would be so inclined.

Within hours I was on the shooting range testing out some of my ideas about the choice of weapon and bullet. Baum wanted a .22 Magnum-caliber bullet, feeling that it would enable a sniper to hit a small target at 100 yards consistently. He then asked for shoulder shots. I disagreed, feeling that the ranges should be shorter, 40 to 60 meters, and the kneecap target that Baum also wanted hit should be expanded to include the leg and hips. I produced a gross anatomy book and argued against aiming at a moving target's shoulder, since the heart and neck were just too close. Viewing the anatomy plates, Baum instantly agreed and we settled in on lower anatomy shots with the kneecap as target zero.

I was against the .22 Magnum because I felt it had too high a signature, producing unwanted and unneeded noise, not to mention higher training costs and less choice of rifles and bullet design. I liked the hypervelocity Remington Yellow Jacket hollowpoint ammo, which I had range-tested against the knee bones of dead steers, finding that the tiny bullet splattered them even at 100 yards. I used an Anschutz single-shot bolt action .22 LR with a Lyman Superspot Target Scope 5X-20X for the initial tests. For our field work and range of operation, I felt the Ruger 10/22 with sound suppressor and 3X-9X multireticle scope would be more than adequate.

Baum came around to the idea. I showed him a slew of books on riot control, sniping, close-quarter fighting, etc. that I'd just ordered from Paladin Press, books that I had poured over and devoured in intense study, including the classic works by the dean of the profession, Col. Rex Applegate. With these in hand, we were ready to enter the mouth of a riot to learn how it worked Arab style.

1982: Riot in Ramallah

A very noisy and violent series of riots were taking place in Ramallah, a small town north of Jerusalem. Some of the

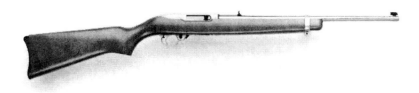

THE RUGER 10/22 CARBINE: *The gun I recommended as the instrument to break the Intifada.*

activity was spurred on from a nearby Arab village. We drove into the village in a covered pick-up truck, and I set about peering at the riot through the eyes of the rifle telescope. For this task, I was more interested in learning how the riots were controlled and by whom than in drilling Yellow Jacket holes into kneecaps.

As we drove around the street littered with rocks, bottles, and metal bars, we found ourselves constantly coming into view of road blocks set up with huge rocks, barrels, and burning tires. I noticed right away that the frontline cadres of rioters were made up mostly of women and children. This I felt was very clever on their part. This was excellent propaganda since these riots were not about job losses, alleged racism, and all the usual reasons given by rioters in North America. These riots were instead aimed at causing a pullout of Israeli forces and thus changing the political map of the Mideast. The use of women and children was a brilliant form of psychological warfare, which would place the Israeli army and the police on the defense.

I noticed that behind the front lines there stood one or two men who looked like leaders. They seemed to be in control of orchestrating the riot. I later found out that many of these men were school teachers who were political activists for the cause of the PLO. In these particular riots they always seemed to stay far behind the front lines, using the women and children as cover.

The Camera Weapon

Cameras began to surface among the rioters, and I soon realized that in time, the use of still and video cameras would revolutionize our perception of riots. What they filmed and taped would appear on TV news around the globe. These cameras allowed just about anyone to film and edit a controlled riot any way they deemed fit. Even if the area was closed to the working press, the film and tape would leak to the outside world. What I was watching through my rifle scope was the budding of a technique that would utilize the media to an extent never seen before. The age of the super-controlled mass-media riot had dawned.

Some Notes on the Riot

At times I saw the mob whip itself up into such a frenzy that some literally struck out in anger at their own compatriots. This was something that had been reported to me before, but now, for the first time, I saw the psychology of a frenzied mob at work. Woe be on to anyone falling into the hands of such a mob. I believe no one could survive such an ordeal. We would have to be very careful to protect our men.

Viewing the antics of the rioters through a rifle telescope, I soon realized that kneecap shots were not going to be very easy to pull off. The idea of shots anywhere below the belly button was much more feasible. Kneecap hits were the goal, but one that would be difficult to achieve.

The use of women and children would also pose a psychological problem. It soon became obvious to me that the riot leaders were the prime targets of any deterrent campaign of accurate fire. Ideas that had been theory in discussion now seemed to be clarified in the black smoke of the riot.

When we got back that evening we had much to discuss. Baum's idea of using highly trained specialists was becoming more and more appreciated, as we realized that using regular troops only played into the hands of the rioters who were being manipulated and orchestrated as a "media happening" with the world as the audience. Baum's fear that this would explode in our faces if it appeared on prime time TV around the world was correct.

I realized that normal methods of riot control would not suffice. The snipers had to be used in a way that prohibited their being filmed. The special antiriot troops that would be under our command had to come up with answers that would stop the rioting and yet wouldn't fall into the propaganda trap that was being set. We knew our actions would be viewed as being "fascistic" by the media. We could do no right. The mere fact that the media thought it normal for women and children to be used as cannon fodder proved that point. We had to be careful not to be set up and then pushed into a propaganda trap.

The Best Laid Plans of Mice and Men

We had put together the planning elements needed to form the special unit which would be under the senior supervision of Baum, who would be backed by the then Defense Minister Arik Sharon. Suddenly, everything went haywire. In Damur, Lebanon, the Christians, who had seen thousands of their family members butchered and 9,000 of their women raped by the PLO, took revenge when they captured the PLO camps of Sabra and Shatilla. Tens of thousands of leftists in Israel blamed Sharon in what can only be called a convoluted twisting of the facts, and he was forced to resign. With Arik, as his men affectionately called him, went all hope of implementing the idea of the special units against the upcoming Intifada. When it did arrive, it lasted for more than 72 hours and went on for years. Thousands on both sides were killed and maimed. How much more humane the work of the special unit would have been. Alas, it was not to be, and the rest, as they say, is history.

STREET SURVIVAL LESSON

1) *Propaganda*. Some riots are controlled by riot leaders who cleverly use tactics such as placing women and children into the forefront of the riot so that the media will photograph police or soldiers using force against them. Anyone working in riot control must take this reality into consideration.

SUMMING IT ALL UP

Working with individuals who are constantly under the threat of brutal annihilation by bloodthirsty enemies has given me and my compatriots an excellent perspective on what really works out there in the street. A lifetime of survival experiences have been packed into each year of our survival here. Each of those practical lessons and tricks of the trade can and have spelled the difference between life or death.

What I have written is not the end of the list; the lessons of street survival are constantly being expanded upon. Nor are these lessons the only way to go. There is no ultimate wisdom in survival since the dangers we all face are evolving and changing and we must adapt to them, conquer them, or perish. All wisdom, ideas, and techniques are part of the flow of life. Adapt and modify them as needed to your own street survival needs. In the end, you must make the choice "to be or not to be."